Ketogenic Ninja Foodi Cookbook

Delicious, Simple and Quick Keto Ninja Foodi Recipes For Smart People

Table of Contents

Introduction

The Ninja Foodi is a versatile cooking tool that works as a pressure cooker, a sauté pan, a slow cooker, a broiler, an air fryer, and a food dehydrator, all in one compact package. The pot's multi-function versatility and its unrivaled ability to prepare delicious dishes in an amazingly short time makes it the perfect companion for a time-crunched lifestyle.

This cookbook combines in one place the best of the Ninja Foodi world, giving you a broad selection of flavorful meal choices to lead you to a healthier, happier life on the ketogenic diet.

Ninja Foodi Cooking and Nutrition: Maximizing Your Macronutrient Balance

You've learned how a Ninja Foodi can help you to prepare healthy meals within a minimum of time and fuss, but to fully understand the potential health benefits of pressure cooking and air frying, you need to more fully understand how your body processes the foods you eat. Basic nutritional knowledge begins with understanding the nature of fats, proteins and carbs--the main nutrients you'll see identified in the nutritional information of most foods and recipes.

Fats, proteins, and carbohydrates are compounds called macronutrients. They are categories of substances that fuel our metabolic processes, and we need large amounts of them in order to live. In various combinations, these three types of macronutrients make up most of the foods we eat.

Carbohydrates (or "carbs" for short) make up the bulk of the foods in the typical Western diet. They are chemical compounds that contain carbon, hydrogen, and oxygen, and as we have already learned, they're easily processed by the body into cell-fueling glucose. Common carbohydrates include the fructose sugar in fruits, the lactose sugar in dairy products, and the sucrose in common table sugar. The starches and cellulose in vegetables are also carbohydrates.

Proteins are compounds made up of chains of amino acids. They are not as easily used by the body for fuel, but they are vital for other cell functions, maintenance, and repair. In our diet, proteins primarily come from animal products such as meat or eggs, but they can also be found in some plant-based foods such as nuts and legumes.

Fats are compounds consisting of chains of fatty acids. As a nutrient, fats are an excellent source of energy, but under typical metabolic conditions, they're more often used as a way to store energy for later use. Fatty acids are stored in specialized tissues in the body, and they're only used for energy when necessary. In the diet, fats can come from either animal or plant sources.

To achieve optimal nutrition, you need to eat foods that have the right balance of fats, protein and carbohydrates. Many popular diets, emphasize one category of macronutrient or another, encouraging you to eat more of one and less of the others. The popular ketogenic diet, for example, strives to eliminate most carbohydrates from the diet, instead depending mostly on fats and protein. In general, however, nutritionists usually recommend that you get most of your daily calories from carbohydrates and fats and a smaller proportion of your calories from proteins.

Whatever diet you've chosen to follow (or that your healthcare provider or nutritionist has recommended for you), you'll be best off if you pay attention to the balance of macronutrients in the foods you eat. That's why we've included nutritional information, including proportions of macronutrients, along with each recipe in this book. Be aware that the numbers we've provided are only an estimate, and in actuality they'll vary depending on the exact ingredients you use and the serving size you eat, but we've given you a place to start as you begin to cook and eat more mindfully.

The Ketogenic Diet

In the most basic sense, a ketogenic diet is a nutritional approach that emphasizes relatively high fat intake, moderate protein intake, and low carbohydrate intake. The ultimate goal of the diet is to force the dieter's body to burn fat as fuel instead of carbohydrates, which are the fuel that the metabolic system leans on most heavily under normal, non-ketogenic conditions. The theory is that the body will become used to burning fat stores--and hence begin to produce weight loss--instead of relying on carbohydrate for fuel and storing fat in the body.

Triggering of Ketosis

Usually, the human body generates energy by metabolically converting carbohydrates in food into glucose and then burning the resulting glucose in its cells. Carbohydrates are converted into glucose relatively easily by the body to convert into glucose, so they're an ideal fuel source. The body's metabolic system will rely on carbs when it can, fueling itself with them as they enter the digestive system from food. Stored fat is left in place because it's not needed.

When a person consumes excess carbohydrates, the metabolic system converts any carbs it doesn't need for fuel into fat, which is then stored in various places in the body. The body then resists burning that stored fat, opting instead to burn newly consumed carbs. And the cycle starts over again.

However, if an adequate amount of carbohydrates aren't present in a person's diet, the body will be forced to find other options for the energy it needs. After carbs, the body's next most-preferred fuel source is fat, which is metabolized in the liver. The liver turns fat into fatty acids and other water-soluble molecules called ketone bodies, which can be used in the body's cells as a fuel source. When the liver is actively metabolizing fat and the level of ketone bodies in the blood stream is elevated above typical levels, the body is said to have entered a state of ketosis.

What are the Benefits of a Ketogenic Diet?

Weight loss
The possibility of rapid, dramatic weight loss is the lure of the keto diet for many dieters. It's not uncommon for a keto diet to result in weight loss of several pounds in the first week or so. It's difficult to resist the possibility to such a quick result.

Everyone who adopts a keto diet will experience something different, however. Consistent, sustained weight loss will only happen when the dieter pays careful attention to food intake and follows an exercise program.

Blood Sugar Control

A keto diet can help to eliminate spikes in blood sugar levels by giving your body fats and proteins to process instead of carbs. These nutrients are not as easily or quickly converted to glucose, so blood sugar spikes are not nearly as likely to occur when you eat more fats and proteins and fewer carbs.

Appetite Control

A keto diet can help to stabilize your appetite and eliminate cravings by reducing the ups and downs caused by high carb intake. A diet high in fats and proteins will help you to feel full faster and hold off hunger longer than a diet that relies too heavily on carbohydrates.

Energy Levels

Another benefit of stabilized blood sugar is the stabilization of your energy level throughout the day. When your blood sugar level plummets,, you not only get hungry, you also get tired. Without carbs to provide quick and easy energy, your body doesn't think it has any way to find energy, so it simply gives up and gets lethargic until it convinces you to eat more carbs.

Your body on a keto diet knows it has other options. After you've trained your body to enter a state of ketosis, it knows where to look for energy when there are no carbs readily available. There's plenty of energy to be found in your stored fat, and a body that's used to a keto diet is able to utilize that energy to keep you from feeling tired and lethargic even between meals.

Keto Diet and Insulin Resistance

Insulin is a hormone that allows your body to process glucose. Your body's production of insulin is a natural process that is crucial to controlling the level of glucose in your blood and fueling your cells. Some people, however, develop insulin resistance. That means that insulin becomes less effective at processing glucose in their bodies, leading to elevated blood sugar levels and potentially serious health problems.

A keto diet helps to moderate the problems of insulin resistance by stabilizing blood sugar levels. Your body becomes less dependent on insulin production, and the impact of insulin resistance is decreased, too.

Using the Ninja Foodi on the Keto Diet

What is the Ninja Foodi?

The Ninja Foodi is an extremely versatile cooking appliance that combines the capabilities of a pressure cooker, a slow cooker, a sauté pan, and more into a single device. It and other similar appliances are enjoying a surge in popularity as home chefs are discovering the benefits of pressure cooking and air frying for the first time.

Benefits of Pressure Cooking

The convenience, time- and effort-saving advantages of pressure cooking are one things, but we'll also argue that pressure-cooked foods may even be healthier for you than conventionally cooked foods and that pressure cooking can also be a money saver. We'll even go so far as to say that pressure cooking is good for the environment. Don't believe us? Read on for an explanation.

Pressure cooked foods can be healthier than their conventionally cooked counterparts. Conventional cooking methods are sometimes very destructive to the nutritional content of foods. Cooking methods that use lots of water can leach nutrients from foods, and high temperatures and long cooking times can chemically convert nutrients into less nutritious forms. Pressure cooking, with its lower moisture requirements, relatively low temperatures and short cooking times, can help foods to retain nutrients.

Pressure cooking saves time. This is probably the most important benefit for most pressure-cooking fans. Using a pressure cooker can reduce cooking time for some dishes as much as 70% over conventional cooking methods. That's a huge win for busy people who don't have time to slave over a hot stove for hours. Many pressure-cooker recipes (including many in this book) are one-pot dishes that you can throw together quickly and then go about your business while they cook in a fraction of the time that you might expect.

Pressure cooking saves effort. This benefit is arguably in a close second-place finish in terms of how awesome pressure cooking is. Not only do quick, one-pot recipes save you lots of time when it comes to meal preparation and time spent actively cooking, but the self-contained nature of pressure cookers means that you've got less clean up to do after you've finished eating. That makes the entire cooking process even easier on you, but it is also easier on the environment, which we'll go into below.

Pressure cooking saves energy. Yes, pressure cooking saves energy, and not just yours. An electric pressure cooker generally uses less energy than multiple burners on an electric or gas range or an oven. The pressure cooker has to generate less heat, and its shorter cooking time means that it's turned on for a shorter amount of time.

A less obvious benefit is that a pressure cooker doesn't heat up your kitchen as much as a range or oven does, so your air conditioner doesn't have to work as hard to keep the room cool.

And the one-pot convenience of pressure cooking also translates into less energy expended on clean up, including hot water generation and the energy required to run you dishwasher.

All of these energy-saving benefits result in some actual cost saving for you and some helpful resource conservation for the planet.

Benefits of Air Frying

The most obvious benefit of using an air fryer is that it allows you to get the delicious crispiness of fried foods while using much less oil or fat than you'd need to use for conventional frying. The result is that air-fried foods typically have fewer calories, less cholesterol, and less harmful fat.

Air fryers also often use less energy than conventional frying techniques, are quicker, and are easier to clean up.

Ninja Foodi Features

A Ninja Foodi can function as a stand-alone electric pressure cooker that operates essentially the same way (although typically at a lower pressure) than a traditional stove-top pressure cooker.

Ninja Foodis also have non-pressure-cooking modes, including a Sauté mode, a Broil mode, and a Dehydrate mode. In the saute mode, the inner liner of the pot heats to a relatively high heat so that foods can be browned or sautéed directly in the pot. This mode can also be used to reheat sauces and dishes when necessary after the end of a pressure-cooking cycle.

Ninja Foodis also feature a low-heat, no-pressure slow cooker mode. This mode is designed to cook dishes at a low temperature over a long period of time.

Ninja Foodis also include steamer racks so that you can steam vegetables or other dishes directly in the pot.

Ninja Foodi Controls

The controls on individual Ninja Foodi models vary along the product line, but all models include controls to activate and adjust a range of cooking modes, as well as a group of standard basic controls. To learn how to use your Foodi, and to learn how to operate the unit safely, refer to the user manual that came with the unit.

Most Foodi models are equipped with the controls we've listed below, but you should consult your unit's manual to see which controls and accessories your Foodi is equipped with.

Function Controls

Pressure: This button puts the Ninja Foodi into a pressure-cooking mode. Use this mode to cook food relatively quickly and to retain as much moisture in the food as possible.

Steam: This button initiates the steam-cooking mode. Use it to gently cook foods such as tender vegetables at a high temperature.

Slow Cook: Use this mode to cook foods gently at relatively low temperature over a long period of time.

Sear/Sauté: This button puts the Foodi into saute mode, turning the pot into something similar to a skillet. Use it to brown food or to heat or simmer sauces.

Air Crisp: This button starts the air-fryer mode. Use it to make foods crispy using very little or no oil.

Bake/Roast: Use this mode to roast or bake foods as if the Foodi were an oven.

Broil: This button initiates a mode that will brown or caramelize foods.

Dehydrate: This mode uses heat and air circulation to remove moisture from foods. This function is not available on all models.

Operation Controls

TEMP buttons: These up and down arrow buttons allow you to adjust the cooking temperature after you've selected a cooking mode.

TIME buttons: These arrow buttons allow to adjust the cooking time after you've entered a cooking mode.

START/STOP button: This button begins a cooking cycle after the mode, temperature and time have been selected. Pushing the button again during a cooking cycle stops the cycle.

KEEP WARM: After a cooking cycle, the Foodi will automatically revert to a keep-warm mode to keep food at serving temperature. The keep-warm mode will shut off automatically after 12 hours, or you can end it at any time by pushing this button.

POWER: This button turns the unit on and off. Pushing it during a cooking cycle will automatically end the cycle.

Ninja Foodi Accessories

Cooking Pot: This main cooking pot is the vessel you'll use to cook most foods using the pressure mode. Unless otherwise specified, the recipes in this book make use of the main cooking pot.

Cooking Rack: This reversible rack is used to keep food from touching the base of the pot and can be reversed to raise food to two different levels. The rack is typically used when steaming foods, to keep the food elevated above the liquid in the pot that's generating steam.

Crisping Lid: This hinged lid is used during Air Crisp, sauté, broil and bake cooking modes.

Air Crisp (Cook & Crisp) Basket: This basket fits inside the cooking pot and is used during Air Crisp cooking cycles.

Pressure Lid: This secondary lid fits over the pot and is used during pressure- and steam-cooking cycles. It is equipped with a pressure release valve and must be locked in place during pressure and steam cooking cycles. Read your manual carefully to learn you to use the pressure lid, and always follow all safety guidelines while you're using it.

Pressure Release

At the end of a pressure-cooking cycle, the steam pressure inside the Ninja Foodi must be vented. You can release the pressure manually immediately following the cooking cycle, or you can allow the pot to vent naturally and gradually through the steam release valve. A slow natural release of pressure may cause some foods to overcook, and many recipes in this book will direct you to release the pressure manually as soon as the cooking cycle is finished.

Manual (Quick) Release: To vent the pot's pressure manually, turn the steam release handle to the VENT position until the float valve drops, being careful not to get your hands, face, or any other exposed part of your body in the way of escaping steam. Never pull the steam release handle out when the pot is under pressure, and move the handle back to the Sealing position immediately if food splatters through the valve.

Natural Release: If you don't do a manual release at the end of the cooking cycle, pressure will begin to vent naturally through the release valve. A full release of pressure may take as long as 40 minutes. Many recipes in this book will direct you to allow the pot to vent naturally for a specified period of time, after which you should release any remaining pressure manually.

Ninja Foodi Safety

Before operating your Ninja Foodi, read the included operation manual completely so that you thoroughly understand the proper way to use and maintain the appliance.

Always be sure that the pot is properly covered, sealed and locked before you initiate any pressure-cooking cycle. Always check to be sure that the sealing ring is clean, undamaged and in place on the underside of the pot cover before sealing the pot at the start of a cooking cycle.

Always add at least 4 ounces (8 ounces for steam cooking) of water-based (not oil-based) liquid to the pot to ensure that there is enough liquid to generate steam during a pressure cooking cycle. Never, however, fill the pot above the PRESSURE MAX line.

Take extreme care during and after any pressure-cooking cycle, even if the cycle is interrupted before it finishes. The pressure inside the pot can cause very hot steam or other contents to escape through the float valve if the pot is improperly sealed or if the steam release handle is opened. Never open the pot cover before the pressure inside the pot is completely released.

When venting pressure at the end of a cooking cycle, keep your hands and face away from the valve. Escaping steam is extremely hot and can cause serious burns to exposed skin.

Keep the float valve clean and free of food debris. If the float valve is stuck, vent all the pressure from the pot and then free the stuck valve using a pencil, the handle of wooden spoon, or a similar utensil.

Recipes

Eating a healthy diet requires most of us who haven't been eating mindfully to make some major changes to the way we eat. That can be a challenge, especially for busy people who don't have the time to learn a whole new way of menu and meal planning. The convenience of the Ninja Foodi, however, makes it much easier to stick to a diet that can improve your health and lifestyle.

The recipes we've included here use the Ninja Foodi's unique features to get the most from the foods that fall within the boundaries of a healthy diet, allowing you to have a different and delicious dish every day of the week. And the simplicity of the recipes, coupled with the quick cook times of the Ninja Foodi, ensures that anyone, no matter how pressed for time, can fit a healthy diet into their lifestyle, no matter how busy they are or how little time that they have for cooking.

Breakfast

A Ninja Foodi is well-suited to making quick work of traditional breakfast foods like eggs and bacon, but your pressure-cooker breakfast doesn't have to be constrained to the basics. These breakfast recipes will give you new takes on old favorites so you can begin each day in a delectable way. In fact, a Ninja Foodi is the ideal assistant for busy people who need a nutritious breakfast (hint: that's all of us). With only a little planning and a miniscule amount of effort ahead of time, you can have a satisfying and fortifying breakfast every single day.

Ninja Foodi Cauliflower Hashbrown Bake

Servings: 12
Time Required: 35 minutes
Ingredients:

- 6 eggs, beaten
- 30 oz. grated cauliflower
- ¼ cup milk
- 1 large onion, chopped
- 3 Tbsp. olive oil
- 1 lb. cooked ham, cubed
- ½ cup cheddar cheese

Method:

1. Turn your Foodi's on sauté mode.
2. Add olive oil and chopped onion and sauté until translucent.
3. Add cauliflower. Set Air Crisp to 350 degrees for 15 minutes. Flip the mixture after about 8 minutes.
4. Mix together eggs and milk. Pour over the mixture and add the cubed ham.
5. Set Foodi to Air Crisp at 350 degrees for 10 minutes. Cook until the eggs are set and the top is golden brown.
6. Top with cheddar cheese and close lid until cheese is melted, approximately one minute.

Nutrition Information Per Serving:

- Total Fat: 14 grams
- Carbohydrates: 8 grams
- Protein: 14 grams

Ninja Foodi Soft-Boiled Eggs

Servings: 6

Time Required: About 5 minutes

Ingredients:

- 6 large eggs
- ¾ cup water

Method:

1. Put the steamer rack into the Ninja Foodi and pour in the water.
2. Place eggs, still in the shell, on top of the steamer rack.
3. Cover and lock the pot.
4. Using the Steam function, adjust the cook time to 2 minutes.
5. When the cook time is up, remove the eggs and serve hot.
6. Serves six.

Nutrition Information Per Serving:

- Total Fat: 5 grams
- Carbohydrates: 0 gram
- Protein: 6 grams

Ninja Foodi Omelet Cups

Servings: 4
Time Required: About 15 minutes
Ingredients:

- 4 eggs
- ½ cup onion, diced
- ½ cup bell pepper, diced
- ½ cup cheddar cheese, grated
- ¼ cup half and half

Method:

1. In a mixing bowl, whisk together all ingredients until the eggs are beaten and everything is well combined. Season with salt and pepper.
2. Divide the mixture between four small canning jars. Loosely screw the lids onto the jars.
3. Place a steamer rack in the Ninja Foodi and pour 2 cups water into the pot.
4. Place the jars on the steamer rack.
5. Cover and lock the pot.
6. Using the Steam mode, set the cook time for 5 minutes.
7. At the end of the cook time, carefully vent the pot manually.
8. Remove the jars from the pot and serve the eggs in the jars.

Nutrition Information Per Serving:

Total Fat: 9 grams
Carbohydrates: 2 grams
Protein: 9 grams

Ninja Foodi Ham and Egg Breakfast

Servings: 6
Time Required: About 4.5 hours
Ingredients:

- 1 onion, diced
- 2 cups cooked ham, cubed
- 2 cups cheddar cheese, grated
- 10 eggs
- 1 cup whole milk
- 1 tsp. salt
- 1 tsp. pepper

Method:

1. Place ham, onion, and cheese in the Ninja Foodi.
2. In a mixing bowl, whisk together the milk and eggs until the eggs are beaten. Add salt and pepper and stir to mix thoroughly.
3. Poor the egg mixture over the ingredients in the pot.
4. Cover and lock the pot.
5. Using the Slow Cooker mode, adjust to a cook time of 4 hours.
6. At the end of the cook time, dish up the scramble and serve hot.
7. Serves six.

Nutrition Information Per Serving:

- Total Fat: 11 grams
- Carbohydrates: 3 grams
- Protein: 11 grams

Ninja Foodi Bacon, Egg and Cheese Cups

Servings: 4
Time Required: About 20 minutes
Ingredients:

- 4 eggs
- ¼ cup egg whites
- 4 slices bacon, cooked crisp and crumbled
- ½ cup reduced-fat cottage cheese
- ¼ cup heavy cream
- 1 bell pepper, diced
- ½ onion, diced
- 1 cup cheddar cheese, grated
- 1 cup water

Method:

1. Combine eggs and egg whites with cheese, cream and cottage cheese in a food processer or blender. Season with salt and pepper. Blend until the ingredients are well combined and smooth, about 30 seconds to a minute.
2. Place the steamer rack in the pot and add the water.
3. Divide the egg mixture evenly between six small canning jars. Top each jar with equal amounts of pepper, onion and bacon crumbles. Put the lids on each jar, but do not tighten the lids tightly.
4. Cover and lock the Ninja Foodi.
5. Using the Steam setting, set the cook time to 12 minutes.
6. When the cooking time is finished, allow the pot to vent naturally for 10 minutes. After 10 minutes, carefully release any remaining steam, being careful not to burn yourself.
7. After a few minutes of cooling, the cooked eggs should slide out of the jars, or you can serve them in the jars.

Nutrition Information Per Serving:

- Total Fat: 8 grams
- Carbohydrates: 3 grams
- Protein: 9 grams

Ninja Foodi Mini Mushroom Quiche

Servings: 4
Time Required: About 20 minutes
Ingredients:

- ½ cup Swiss cheese, grated
- ¼ cup fresh mushrooms, chopped
- ¼ cup spring onion, diced
- 4 eggs
- ¼ cup milk
- 1 cup water

Method:

1. Using a silicone or heat-proof egg tray, divide the cheese evenly between the cups in the tray, pressing the cheese into the bottom of the cups.
2. Divide the mushrooms and onions among the cups, placing them on top of the cheese.
3. Combine eggs with in a food processor or blender. Season with salt and pepper. Blend until the ingredients are well combined and smooth, about 30 seconds to a minute. Pour the mixture into the cups on top of the cheese, mushrooms and onions.
4. Place the steamer rack in the pot and add the water.
5. Carefully place the tray on top of the steamer rack.
6. Cover and lock the Ninja Foodi.
7. Using the Steam setting, set the cook time to 5 minutes.
8. When the cooking time is finished, allow the pot to vent naturally for 5 minutes. After 5 minutes, carefully release any remaining steam, being careful not to burn yourself.
9. After a few minutes of cooling, pop the mini quiches out of the tray and serve immediately.

Nutrition Information Per Serving:

Total Fat: 8 grams
Carbohydrates: 3 grams
Protein: 9 grams

Soups and Stews

When you cook soups and stews in the Ninja Foodi, the pot does most of the work. With many of these recipes, all you'll have to do is dump the ingredients into the pot and start a cooking cycle. In a very short time, you'll have a delicious, richly flavored soup.

That doesn't mean, though, that you'll have a *boring* soup. We've included a collection of soup recipes that take advantage of the spices and ingredients of international cuisine to keep your daily menu exciting. The recipes range from the ultra-traditional--things like chicken soup and chili--to the exotic. We've included flavors from East Asia, India, Mexico and more, so whatever you're in the mood for, you'll be able to find it here. And if you're in the mood to try something totally new, we're pretty sure you can find *that* here, too.

Ninja Foodi Cheesy Cauliflower Soup

Servings: 10
Time Required: About 45 minutes
Ingredients:

- 1 head cauliflower, chopped
- ½ onion, chopped
- 2 Tbsp. olive oil
- 3 cups chicken stock
- 1 tsp. garlic powder
- 1 tsp. kosher salt
- 4 oz. cream cheese, cubed
- 1 cup cheddar cheese, grated
- ½ cup milk

Method:

1. Press the sauté button and add olive oil to pot. Add onion and cook until softened, about 3 minutes.
2. Add cauliflower, stock, salt and garlic powder.
3. Cover the pot and cook on Pressure setting for 5 minutes.
4. Vent the pot and remove the cover.
5. Transfer cauliflower to a blender or food processor and blend to a smooth puree.
6. Set the pot to the "Keep Warm" setting. Return pureed cauliflower to the pot and add the cream cheese and cheddar cheese, stirring as the mixture heats.
7. When the cheese has melted, add the milk and heat thoroughly.
8. Serves four.

Nutrition Information Per Serving

- Total Fat: 8 grams
- Carbohydrates: 17 grams
- Protein: 5 grams

Ninja Foodi Ranch Chicken and Cheese Soup

Servings: 10

Time Required: About 35 minutes

Ingredients:

- 2 chicken breasts, boneless and skinless, cooked and cubed
- 3 cups chicken stock
- ½ cup celery, diced
- ¼ cup diced onion
- 1 clove garlic, minced
- 1 Tbsp. butter
- 1 cup heavy cream
- 2 cups cheddar cheese, grated
- 1 Tbsp. ranch dressing mix
- ¼ tsp. red pepper flakes

Method:

1. Combine all ingredients, excluding the heavy cream and the cheddar cheese, in the Ninja Foodi.
2. Using the Pressure setting, cook for 10 minutes under high pressure.
3. At the end of the cook time, carefully vent the pot manually.
4. Slowly stir in the cream and cheese, stirring until the cheese is melted.
5. Transfer from the pot to serving bowls and serve hot.

Nutrition Information Per Serving:

- Total Fat: 10 grams
- Carbohydrates: 6 grams
- Protein: 12 grams

Ninja Foodi Low-Carb Chili

Servings: 10
Time Required: About an hour
Ingredients:

- 2 ½ lb. ground beef, 85 percent lean
- ½ large white onion, diced
- 8 cloves garlic, minced
- 2 cans (15 oz. each) diced tomatoes, liquid reserved
- 6 oz. tomato paste
- 4 oz. canned green chilis, liquid reserved
- 2 Tbsp. Worcestershire sauce
- ¼ cup chili powder
- 2 Tbsp. cumin
- 1 Tbsp. dried oregano
- 2 tsp. kosher salt
- 1 tsp. freshly ground black pepper
- 1 Tbsp. olive oil

Method:

1. Press the Sauté button on the pot and add oil. When the oil is hot, add the onions to the pot and sauté until soft and translucent, about 5 minutes.
2. Add garlic to the pot and sauté for one minute more.
3. Add ground beef to the pot and sauté until the meat is thoroughly browned, stirring constantly with a wooden spoon or spatula. This should take about 10 minutes.
4. Add the rest of the ingredients to the pot and stir to combine.
5. Cover and lock the pot and stop the Sauté cycle.
6. Push the Pressure button and cook for 30 minutes.
7. When the cooking time is finished allow the pot to vent naturally.
8. After the pressure is fully vented, remove the pot cover and transfer the chili to serving bowls.

Nutrition Information Per Serving:

- Total Fat: 18 grams
- Carbohydrates: 13 grams
- Protein: 23 grams

Ninja Foodi Creamy Green Chili Soup

Servings: 10
Time Required: About 45 minutes
Ingredients:

- 2 lb. ground beef, 85 percent lean
- ¼ cup onion, diced
- 4 cloves garlic, minced
- 2 Tbsp. chili powder
- 2 tsp. cumin
- 20 oz. canned diced tomatoes
- 4 oz. canned green chilis
- 32 oz. beef stock
- 8 oz. cream cheese
- ½ cup heavy cream
- 1 Tbsp. olive oil

Method:

1. Press the Sauté button on the pot and add oil. When the oil is hot, add the onions to the pot and sauté until soft and translucent, about 5 minutes.
2. Add garlic to the pot and sauté for one minute more.
3. Add ground beef to the pot and sauté until the meat is thoroughly browned, stirring constantly with a wooden spoon or spatula. This should take about 10 minutes.
4. Add the rest of the ingredients, excluding the cream and cream cheese, to the pot and stir to combine.
5. Cover and lock the pot and stop the Sauté cycle.
6. Push the Pressure button and adjust cook time to 5 minutes.
7. When the cooking time is finished allow the pot to vent naturally for 10 minutes.
8. After 10 minutes, carefully vent any remaining steam and remove lid.
9. Stir in cream and cream cheese, stirring constantly until cream cheese is melted and soup is thick and creamy.
10. Transfer to serving bowls and serve hot.

Nutrition Information Per Serving:

- Total Fat: 28 grams
- Carbohydrates: 8 grams
- Protein: 27 grams

Ninja Foodi Chinese Chicken Soup

Servings: 10
Time Required: About an hour
Ingredients:

- 1 lb. chicken breast, boneless and skinless, cut into bite-size pieces
- 1 Tbsp. peanut butter
- 1 Tbsp. black bean paste
- 2 tsp. soy sauce
- 2 tsp. rice wine vinegar
- ½ tsp. freshly ground black pepper
- ¼ cup water

Method:

1. In a medium bowl, combine peanut butter, bean paste, soy sauce, vinegar, pepper and water.
2. Add chicken and toss to coat. Allow the chicken to marinate for 30 minutes.
3. Put everything into the Ninja Foodi, along with another ½ cup water.
4. Cover and lock the pot.
5. Using the Pressure mode, cook for 7 minutes.
6. At the end of the cooking time, allow the pot to vent naturally for 10 minutes. After 10 minutes, release any remaining pressure and uncover the pot.
7. Transfer to serving bowls and serve garnished with chopped fresh cilantro.

Nutrition Information Per Serving:

- Total Fat: 7 grams
- Carbohydrates: 7 grams
- Protein: 22 grams

Ninja Foodi Spicy Thai Pork Soup

Servings: 10
Time Required: About 45 minutes
Ingredients:

- 1 lb. pork shoulder, cut into bite-size pieces
- 2 Tbsp. soy sauce
- 2 Tbsp. rice vinegar
- 2 tsp. Thai chili peppers, chopped
- 1 tsp. salt
- 6 cloves garlic, minced
- 3-inch piece of fresh ginger, peeled and minced
- ½ onion, sliced
- 2 Tbsp. olive oil
- 2 Tbsp. black bean paste
- 3 cups water

Method:

1. Press the Sauté button on the Ninja Foodi and heat the oil in the pot. When the oil is hot, add the ginger and garlic, and sauté until fragrant, about a minute.
2. Stop the Sauté cycle.
3. Add all the other ingredients to the pot, stirring to combine.
4. Cover and lock the pot.
5. Using the Pressure mode, cook at high pressure for 20 minutes.
6. At the end of the cook time, allow the pot to vent naturally for 10 minutes. After 10 minutes, carefully vent any remaining steam and uncover the pot.
7. Transfer the soup to serving bowls and serve hot, garnished with chopped fresh cilantro.

Nutrition Information Per Serving:

Total Fat: 8 grams
Carbohydrates: 7 grams
Protein: 10 grams

Ninja Foodi Broccoli Cheese Soup

Servings: 10
Time Required: About 35 minutes
Ingredient:

- 1 cup broccoli, chopped
- 5 oz. cheddar cheese, grated
- 2 Tbsp. butter
- ¼ cup onion, diced
- ¼ cup celery, diced
- 1 ½ cups chicken stock
- ½ cup heavy cream
- 1 Tbsp. olive oil

Method:

1. Press the Sauté button on the pot and add oil. When the oil is hot, add the onions and celery to the pot and sauté until the onion is soft and translucent, about 5 minutes.
2. Add garlic to the pot and sauté for one minute more.
3. Add the rest of the ingredients, excluding the cream and cheese, to the pot and stir to combine.
4. Cover and lock the pot and stop the Sauté cycle.
5. Push the Pressure button and adjust cook time to 5 minutes.
6. When the cooking time is finished, allow the pot to vent naturally for 10 minutes.
7. After 10 minutes, carefully vent any remaining steam and remove lid.
8. Stir in cream, stirring constantly until the cheese is melted and soup is thick and creamy.
9. Transfer to serving bowls and serve hot.

Nutrition Information Per Serving:

- Total Fat: 36 grams
- Carbohydrates: 5 grams
- Protein: 13 grams

Ninja Foodi Green Chili Chicken Soup

Servings: 10
Time Required: About an hour
Ingredients:

- ½ cup dry navy beans, soaked for an hour in hot water
- 1 onion diced
- 3 New Mexico green chili peppers, chopped
- 5 cloves garlic, minced
- 1 cup cauliflower, diced
- 1 lb. chicken breast, boneless and skinless, cut into bite-size pieces
- ¼ cup fresh cilantro, chopped
- 1 tsp. ground coriander
- 1 tsp. ground cumin
- 1 tsp. salt
- 2 oz. cream cheese

Method:

1. Put all the ingredients, excluding the cream cheese, into your Ninja Foodi.
2. Cover and lock the pot.
3. Using the Pressure mode, cook for 15 minutes.
4. At the end of the cooking time, allow the pot to vent naturally for 10 minutes. After 10 minutes, carefully release any remaining steam and uncover the pot.
5. Transfer the chicken to a plate and set aside.
6. Using an immersion blender, blend the soup until it is smooth.
7. Press the Sauté button on the pot and allow the soup to reheat.
8. When the soup is bubbly, stir in the cream cheese until it's melted.
9. Return the chicken to the soup and stir until everything is heated through.
10. Transfer the soup to serving bowls and serve hot.

Nutrition Information Per Serving:

- Total Fat: 5 grams
- Carbohydrates: 13 grams
- Protein: 22 grams

Ninja Foodi Cream of Squash Soup

Servings: 10
Time Required: About 45 minutes
Ingredients:

- 10 cups butternut squash, cubed
- 1 Tbsp. olive oil
- 1 onion, chopped
- 4 cloves garlic, minced
- 1 ½ tsp. salt
- ½ tsp. black pepper
- 5 cups vegetable stock
- 1 cup heavy cream

Method:

1. Press the sauté button on the Ninja Foodi and add oil. Add onion, garlic, salt and pepper and sauté, stirring, until the onion is translucent.
2. Add squash and stock to the pot. Cover and lock the pot.
3. Press the Pressure button and set cook time to 10 minutes.
4. At the end of the cook time, carefully vent the pot.
5. Uncover the pot and add the cream, stirring to combine. If you have an immersion blender, use it to puree the soup in the pot. If not, transfer the soup to a blender or food processor and blend to a smooth puree.
6. Serve warm. Serves 10.

Nutrition Information Per Serving:

- Total Fat: 22 grams
- Carbohydrates: 9 grams
- Protein: 3 grams

Ninja Foodi Chinese-Style Mushroom Soup

Servings: 10
Time Required: About 45 minutes
Ingredients:

- 5 cups chicken stock
- 1 lb. pork tenderloin or other lean pork, sliced into thin bite-sized pieces
- 1 cup fresh mushrooms, chopped
- 3 Tbsp. soy sauce
- 1 Tbsp. white vinegar
- 2 Tbsp. rice vinegar
- 1 tsp. salt
- 2 tsp. freshly ground black pepper
- 3 Tbsp. water
- 4 eggs, beaten
- 1 lb. tofu, extra firm, cubed

Method:

1. Put all ingredients, excluding eggs and tofu, in the Ninja Foodi.
2. Cover and lock the pot.
3. Using Pressure setting, adjust cook time to 10 minutes. Start cook cycle.
4. At the end of the cooking time, allow the pot to vent naturally for 15 minutes.
5. After 15 minutes, carefully vent any remaining steam and remove the pot cover.
6. Slowly and carefully stir in the tofu and beaten eggs. Allow the warm soup to sit for at least 3 minute to allow the eggs to cook.
7. Transfer to serving bowls and serve hot.

Nutrition Information Per Serving:

Total Fat: 5 grams

Carbohydrates: 5 grams

Protein: 20 grams

Ninja Foodi Yellow Thai Curry

Servings: 10
Time Required: About 35 minutes
Ingredients:

- 4 chicken thighs, skinless boneless, cut into bite-sized pieces
- 14.5-ounce can unsweetened coconut milk, full fat
- 2 teaspoons Thai yellow curry paste
- 2 teaspoons fish sauce
- 3 teaspoons soy sauce
- 1 teaspoon honey
- 2 green onion chopped
- 4 cloves garlic, minced
- 2 tablespoons fresh ginger, minced
- ¼ cup fresh cilantro, chopped
- ¼ cup spring onions, chopped

Method:

1. Place chicken, coconut milk, curry paste, fish sauce, soy sauce and honey into the Ninja Foodi.
2. Cover and lock the pot.
3. Using the Pressure mode, adjust the cook time to 12 minutes. Start the cook cycle.
4. At the end of the cook time, allow the pot to vent naturally for 15 minutes.
5. After 15 minutes, carefully vent any remaining steam and remove the cover.
6. Transfer to serving bowls and garnish with cilantro and spring onions.
7. Serve hot.

Nutrition Information Per Serving:

- Total Fat: 29 grams
- Carbohydrates: 9 grams
- Protein: 14 grams

Ninja Foodi Sausage and Kale Soup

Servings: 10
Time Required: About 30 minutes
Ingredients:

- 4 cups fresh kale, chopped
- ½ lb. smoked sausage, sliced into ½-inch-thick slices
- ½ cup white beans
- 2 cloves garlic, minced
- ½ onion, diced
- ½ cup celery, diced
- ¼ tsp. freshly ground black pepper
- Salt to taste
- 1 cup water

Method:

1. Place all ingredients into your Ninja Foodi.
2. Cover and lock the pot.
3. Using the Pressure mode, cook at high pressure for 8 minutes.
4. At the end of the cook time, allow the pot to vent naturally for 10 minutes.
5. After 10 minutes, carefully vent any remaining steam and remove the cover.
6. Transfer the soup to serving bowls and serve hot.

Nutrition Information Per Serving:

- Total Fat: 15 grams
- Carbohydrates: 15 grams
- Protein: 9 grams

Ninja Foodi Jalapeno Chicken Soup

Servings: 10
Time Required: About 40 minutes
Ingredients:

- 1 lb. boneless skinless chicken breasts, cubed
- 3 Tbsp. butter
- 2 cloves garlic, minced
- ½ onion, chopped
- ½ bell pepper, chopped
- 2 jalapeno peppers, seeded and chopped
- ½ lb. bacon, cooked crisp and crumbled
- 6 oz. cream cheese
- 3 cups chicken stock
- ½ cup heavy cream
- ¼ tsp. paprika
- 1 tsp. cumin
- 1 tsp. salt
- ½ tsp. freshly ground black pepper

Method:

1. Press the sauté button and add butter to the pot. When the butter is melted, add onion, bell pepper and jalapenos and sauté until the onion is soft, about 5 minutes.
2. Add the stock, chicken and cream cheese to the pot, stirring to combine.
3. Cover and lock the pot, and stop the Sauté cycle.
4. Using the Pressure mode, set the cook time to 15 minutes and start the cook cycle.
5. After the cooking time is finished, allow the pot to vent naturally for 5 minutes. After 5 minutes, carefully release any remaining steam and uncover the pot.
6. Stir in the cream and crumbled bacon, stirring to combine.
7. Transfer to serving bowls and serve hot topped with grated cheese.

Nutrition Information Per Serving:

- Total Fat: 40 grams
- Carbohydrates: 4 grams
- Protein: 41 grams

Ninja Foodi Cajun Pork Stew

Servings: 10
Time Required: About 45 minutes
Ingredients:

- 1 onion, chopped
- 4 cloves garlic, minced
- 14 oz. canned diced tomatoes
- 5 oz. canned green chilis
- 1 tsp. dried thyme
- 2 tsp. Cajun seasoning
- 1 lb. pork butt, cubed
- ½ cup heavy whipping cream
- 5 cups baby spinach, chopped

Method:

1. Combine all ingredients except the cream and spinach in the Ninja Foodi.
2. Cover and lock the pot.
3. Using the Pressure mode, set the cook time to 20 minutes, and start the cook cycle.
4. When the cooking cycle is finished, allow the pot to vent naturally for 10 minutes.
5. After 10 minutes, carefully vent any remaining steam and uncover the pot.
6. Press the Sauté button and allow the stew to come to a boil.
7. Stir in the cream, then add the spinach. Cook until the spinach is wilted.
8. Transfer to serving bowls and serve hot.

Nutrition Information Per Serving:

- Total Fat: 17 grams
- Carbohydrates: 9 grams
- Protein: 23 grams

Ninja Foodi Chinese Chicken Soup

Servings: 10
Time Required: About 45 minutes
Ingredients:

- ¼ cup sesame oil
- 6 dried red Thai chilis
- 5 cloves garlic, crushed
- 2 Tbsp. fresh ginger, peeled and sliced
- 2 lb. boneless skinless chicken thighs, chopped
- ¼ cup soy sauce
- ¼ cup dry sherry
- Salt to taste
- ¼ cup fresh Thai basil, chopped

Method:

1. Press the Sauté button and add the oil. Add the garlic, chilis and ginger to the pot and sauté just until fragrant, about a minute.
2. Stop the Sauté cycle and all the other ingredients, excluding the basil, to the pot.
3. Cover and lock the pot.
4. Using the Pressure mode, set the cook time for 7 minutes. Start the cook cycle.
5. At the end of the cooking time, allow the pot to vent naturally for 10 minutes. After 10 minutes, carefully vent any remaining steam and uncover the pot.
6. Press the sauté button again and allow the soup to come to a boil. While the soup heats, stir in the basil.
7. Transfer to serving bowls and serve hot.

Nutrition Information Per Serving:

- Total Fat: 15 grams
- Carbohydrates: 7 grams
- Protein: 31 grams

Ninja Foodi Chicken, Squash and Mushroom Soup

Servings: 10
Time Required: About 30 minutes
Ingredients:

- 1 onion, chopped
- 3 cloves garlic, minced
- 2 cups fresh button mushrooms, chopped
- 1 medium yellow summer squash, chopped
- 1 lb. chicken breast, boneless and skinless, cubed
- 2 cups chicken stock
- Salt and pepper to taste
- 1 tsp. poultry seasoning

Method:

1. Add all ingredients to the Ninja Foodi, then cover and lock the pot.
2. Using the Pressure mode, cook at high pressure for 15 minutes.
3. At the end of the cooking time, allow the pot to vent naturally for 10 minutes.
4. After 10 minutes, carefully vent any remaining steam and uncover the pot.
5. Transfer soup to serving bowls and serve hot.

Nutrition Information Per Serving:

- Total Fat: 15 grams
- Carbohydrates: 9 grams
- Protein: 30 grams

Ninja Foodi Hungarian-Style Goulash

Servings: 10
Time Required: About an hour
Ingredients:

- 1 Tbsp. olive oil
- ½ onion, diced
- 2 cloves of garlic, minced
- 1 lb. ground beef roast, 90 percent lean
- ¼ cup button mushrooms, chopped
- 1 bell pepper, chopped
- ½ cup beef stock
- 1 Tbsp. smoked paprika
- ¼ cup fresh tomatoes, diced
- Salt and pepper to taste

Method:

1. Press the Sauté button on the pot and add oil. When the oil is hot, add the onions to the pot and sauté until soft and translucent, about 5 minutes.
2. Add garlic to the pot and sauté for one minute more.
3. Add ground beef to the pot and sauté until the meat is thoroughly browned, stirring constantly with a wooden spoon or spatula. This should take about 10 minutes.
4. Add the rest of the ingredients to the pot and stir to combine.
5. Cover and lock the pot and stop the Sauté cycle.
6. Push the Pressure button and adjust cook time to 15 minutes.
7. When the cooking time is finished allow the pot to vent naturally for 10 minutes.
8. After 10 minutes, carefully vent any remaining steam and remove lid.
9. Transfer the stew to serving bowls and serve hot garnished with chopped fresh parsley.

Nutrition Information Per Serving:

- Total Fat: 38 grams
- Carbohydrates: 6 grams
- Protein: 20 grams

Ninja Foodi Mexican Beef Stew

Servings: 6
Time Required: About an hour
Ingredients:

- 1 lb. beef chuck steak, cut into large pieces
- 1 onion, chopped
- 1 bell pepper, chopped
- 6 cloves garlic, minced
- 2 cups canned diced tomatoes
- 1 tsp. ground cumin
- 1 tsp. salt
- 1 tsp. smoked paprika
- ½ tsp. red pepper flakes
- ½ tsp. oregano

Method:

1. Put all the ingredients in your Ninja Foodi.
2. Cover and lock the pot.
3. Using the Pressure mode, cook for 30 minutes.
4. At the end of the cooking time, allow the pot to vent naturally for 10 minutes. After 10 minutes, carefully release any remaining steam and uncover the pot.
5. Remove the meat from the sauce and set it aside.
6. Press the Sauté button to begin reheating the sauce.
7. Meanwhile, pull the meat apart into bite-size pieces and return to the sauce.
8. Serve hot with steamed or riced cauliflower.

Nutrition Information Per Serving:

- Total Fat: 13 grams
- Carbohydrates: 11 grams
- Protein: 16 grams

Ninja Foodi Southeast Asian Stew

Servings: 6

Time Required: About 30 minutes

Ingredients:

- 1 lb. beef stew meat
- 1 onion, diced
- 2 Tbsp. tomato paste
- 2 whole star anise
- 1 Tbsp. fresh ginger, peeled and minced
- 3 cloves garlic, minced
- 2 cups water
- 1 tsp. ground pepper
- ½ tsp. Chinese five-spice
- ½ tsp. curry powder
- 2 carrots, peeled and sliced

Method:

1. Place all ingredients in the Ninja Foodi.
2. Cover and lock the pot.
3. Using the Pressure setting, cook for 15 minutes.
4. At the end of the cooking time, allow the pot to vent naturally for 10 minutes. After 10 minutes, carefully release any remaining steam and uncover the pot.
5. Serve the stew hot.

Nutrition Information Per Serving:

- Total Fat: 9 grams
- Carbohydrates: 8 grams
- Protein: 15 grams

Ninja Foodi Red Chili

Servings: 10
Time Required: About 50 minutes
Ingredients:

- 3 tsp. chili powder
- 2 tsp. ground cumin
- 2 tsp. salt
- 1 tsp. dried oregano
- 1 Tbsp. olive oil
- 1 onion, chopped
- 2 cloves garlic, minced
- 1 lb. ground beef, 90 percent lean
- 1 cup canned diced tomatoes
- 1 Tbsp. canned chipotle chilis, chopped
- 2 corn tortillas, torn into small pieces
- ½ cup water

Method:

1. In a small bowl, mix chili powder, cumin, salt and oregano.
2. In a blender or food processor, blend tomatoes, chilis, and tortilla pieces until smooth.
3. Press the Sauté button on the Ninja Foodi and heat the oil in the pot. When the oil is hot, sauté the onions until they're softened, about 3 minutes. Add the garlic and sauté for about a minute more.
4. Add the ground beef to the pot and sauté until it's well browned and broken up.
5. Stir in the spice mixture and sauté until fragrant, about 30 seconds.
6. Add the tomato/tortilla mixture to the pot, along with ½ cup water.
7. Stop the Sauté cycle and cover and lock the pot.
8. Using the Pressure mode, cook for 10 minutes.
9. At the end of the cook time, allow the pot to vent naturally for 10 minutes. After 10 minutes, carefully release any remaining pressure and uncover the pot.
10. Transfer the chili to serving bowls and serve hot.

Nutrition Information Per Serving:

- Total Fat: 24 grams
- Carbohydrates: 12 grams
- Protein: 30 grams

Ninja Foodi Green Chili

Servings: 10
Time Required: About 1.25 hours
Ingredients:

- 2 lb. pork butt, cut into large pieces
- 3 tomatillos, sliced
- 3 jalapeno peppers, seeded and chopped
- 2 New Mexico green chili peppers, seeded and chopped
- 6 cloves garlic, minced
- 1 tomato, chopped
- 2 tsp. cumin
- Salt and pepper to taste

Method:

1. Put the tomatillos, jalapenos, New Mexico chilis, garlic, and tomato into the Ninja Foodi.
2. Put the pork pieces on top of the vegetables in the pot.
3. Add the cumin, salt, and pepper on top of the meat.
4. Cover and lock the pot.
5. Using the Pressure mode, cook for 30 minutes.
6. At the end of the cooking time, allow the pot to vent naturally for 10 minutes. After 10 minutes, release any remaining pressure and uncover the pot.
7. Carefully remove the pieces of meat and set aside on a plate.
8. Using an immersion blender, blend the sauce in the pot until it's smooth.
9. Return the pork to the pot and stir to combine.
10. Transfer the chili to serving bowls and serve hot, garnished with chopped fresh cilantro.

Nutrition Information Per Serving:

- Total Fat: 4 grams
- Carbohydrates: 4 grams
- Protein: 26 grams

Ninja Foodi Tortilla Soup

Servings: 10

Time Required: About 1.25 hours

Ingredients:

- 1 lb. chicken breast, boneless and skinless
- 2 corn tortillas, torn into pieces
- ½ onion, chopped
- 1 cup tomatoes, chopped
- 2 cloves garlic
- 1 Tbsp. canned chipotle chili in adobo sauce, chopped
- ½ jalapeno pepper
- ¼ cup fresh cilantro, chopped
- 1 tsp. salt
- 1 Tbsp. olive oil
- 4 cups water

Method:

1. In a blender or food processor, combine onion, tomatoes, garlic, chipotle, jalapeno and cilantro. Blend until the mixture is smooth.
2. Press the Sauté button on your Ninja Foodi and heat the oil in the pot. When the oil is hot, add the blended mixture to the pot. Cook, stirring, until fragrant, about a minute or two.
3. Add the tortillas, chicken, and water to the pot.
4. Stop the Sauté cycle and cover and lock the pot.
5. Using the Pressure mode, cook for 20 minutes.
6. At the end of the cooking time, allow the pot to vent naturally for 10 minutes. After 10 minutes, carefully vent any remaining steam and uncover the pot.
7. Remove the chicken from the pot and set aside to cool slightly. When it is cool enough to handle, shred it with a fork or your fingers.
8. Return the chicken to the pot and press the Sauté button again. Allow the soup to reheat, then transfer to serving bowls and serve hot.

Nutrition Information Per Serving:

- Total Fat: 5 grams
- Carbohydrates: 5 grams
- Protein: 12 grams

Ninja Foodi Vegetable Soup

Servings: 10
Time Required: About 30 minutes
Ingredients:

- 1 turnip, cut into bite-size pieces
- 1 onion, chopped
- 6 stalks celery, diced
- 1 carrot, sliced
- 15 oz. pumpkin puree
- 1 lb. green beans frozen or fresh
- 8 cups chicken stock
- 2 cups water
- 1 Tbsp. fresh basil, chopped
- ¼ tsp. thyme leaves
- 1/8 tsp. rubbed sage
- Salt to taste
- 1 lb. fresh spinach, chopped

Method:

1. Put all the ingredients, excluding the spinach, into the Ninja Foodi.
2. Cover and lock the pot.
3. Using the Pressure mode, cook for 10 minutes.
4. At the end of the cooking time, allow the pot to vent naturally for 10 minutes. After 10 minutes, carefully vent any remaining steam and uncover the pot.
5. Add the spinach and stir until it's wilted, about 5 minutes.
6. Transfer to serving bowls and serve hot.

Nutrition Information Per Serving

- Total Fat: 0 gram
- Carbohydrates: 10 grams
- Protein: 3 grams

Ninja Foodi Cabbage Soup

Servings: 10
Time Required: About 45 minutes
Ingredients:

- 2 lb. ground beef, 90 percent lean
- ¼ cup onion, diced
- 1 clove garlic, minced
- 1 tsp. cumin
- 1 head cabbage, chopped
- 4 cubes bouillon
- 1 ¼ cup canned diced tomatoes
- 5 oz. canned green chilis
- 4 cups beef stock
- Salt and pepper to taste

Method:

1. Press the Sauté button on the Ninja Foodi and allow the pot to heat. When the pot is hot, add the ground beef and brown the meat, stirring to break it up as it browns. This should take about 10 minutes.
2. When the meat is browned, add the onions and sauté for 5-7 minutes more. Add the garlic and sauté for one more minute.
3. Stop the Sauté cycle.
4. Add the rest of the ingredients to the pot. Cover and lock the pot.
5. Using the Pressure mode, cook for 15 minutes.
6. At the end of the cooking time, carefully vent the pot manually and uncover the pot.
7. Transfer to serving bowls and serve hot.

Nutrition Information Per Serving:

- Total Fat: 18 grams
- Carbohydrates: 6 grams
- Protein: 17 grams

Ninja Foodi Bone Broth

Servings: 10
Time Required: About 2.5 hours
Ingredients:

- 4 lb. chicken parts, including bones, skin and/or fat
- 1 onion, chopped
- 2 carrots, chopped
- 2 stalks celery, chopped
- 2 cloves garlic, peeled and chopped
- 6 sprigs fresh parsley
- 1 Tbsp. cider vinegar
- 1 tsp. sea salt
- 4 quarts water

Method:

1. Add all the ingredients to your Ninja Foodi pressure cooker pot.
2. Cover and lock the pot.
3. Using the Pressure mode, cook for 2 hours.
4. At the end of the cooking time, allow the pot to vent naturally for 15 minutes.
5. After 15 minutes, carefully vent any remaining pressure and uncover the pot.
6. Very carefully use a strainer to remove the solids from the stock.
7. Transfer the broth to clean jars and refrigerate. The broth will keep in the refrigerator for up to 5 days, or you can freeze it in freezer-safe containers for up to 3 months.

Meat and Poultry

Meat and poultry dishes are the centerpiece of most Western diets, but they also are the type of dishes that is most challenging to make interesting day after day. They also tend to require a lot of time and attention to prepare, making them an obstacle for the time-challenged chef. One of the Foodi's most amazing strengths is its ability to cook up meat dishes quickly and with very little fuss.

Don't get us wrong; we've included some very tasty meat and poultry recipes in this book, but we've made it our goal to keep the recipes simple, so that the Ninja Foodi can take the burden off your shoulders.

Ninja Foodi Crispy Mexican-Style Pork

Servings: 4
Time Required: 55 minutes
Ingredients:

- 2 lb. pork butt, cut into 2-inch cubes
- 1 tsp. kosher salt
- ½ tsp. oregano
- ½ tsp. cumin
- 1 yellow onion, peeled and halved
- 6 garlic cloves, minced
- ½ cup chicken broth

Method:

1. Place pork, salt, oregano, and cumin in Ninja Foodi pressure cooker pot and stir to combine, being sure to entirely coat the pork with the seasoning.
2. Mix together the onion, garlic cloves, and chicken broth in a small bowl, then pour the mixture over the pork in the pot.
3. Close and lock the lid. Cook in the Pressure mode at high pressure for 20 minutes.
4. Once the cook time is complete, do a quick release of the pressure. Once all the pressure is released, open the lid and remove the onion, and garlic cloves.
5. Set the Ninja Foodi to sauté and select medium-high. Bring the liquid to a simmer and cook until it reduces by about half, approximately 10-15 minutes.
6. Once half or more of the liquid is gone, stop the sauté cycle and close the Air Crisp lid.
7. Select to Broil for 8 minutes.
8. Serve topped with chopped fresh cilantro

Nutrition Information Per Serving:

- Total Fat: 13 grams
- Carbohydrates: 8 grams
- Protein: 43 grams

Ninja Foodi Roast Chicken

Servings: 4
Time Required: 40 minutes
Ingredients:

- 1 whole chicken (3 1/2-4 lbs)
- 1 cup water
- 4 Tbsp. butter
- 1 tsp. paprika
- 1 tsp. garlic powder
- ½ tsp. onion powder
- 1 tsp. salt
- ¼ cup flour
- 2 cups chicken stock

Method:

1. Wash and pat the chicken dry. Season with salt, pepper, garlic powder and onion powder. Place chicken in the Air Crisp basket.
2. Pour the water into the Foodi's main pot.
3. Place the fryer basket into the main pot.
4. Cook on high pressure for 15 minutes.
5. When cooking time is finished, do a quick release. Remove the chicken and the fryer basket, and discard the liquid from the main pot.
6. Return the chicken and the basket to the main pot.
7. Set to Air Crisp at 400 degrees for 15 minutes, checking occasionally until the chicken is golden brown. Remove the chicken and the basket, and cover with tin foil, allowing the chicken to rest until it reaches an internal temperature of 165 degrees.

Nutrition Information Per Serving:

Total Fat: 8 grams
Carbohydrates: 0 gram
Protein: 22 grams

Ninja Foodi Crispy Breaded Pork Chops

Servings: 6
Time Required: About 15 minutes
Ingredients:

- Olive oil cooking spray
- 6 center cut boneless pork chops, 3/4-inch thick, 5 oz. each
- Kosher salt
- 1 large egg, beaten
- ½ cup panko bread crumbs
- 1/3 cup crushed cornflake cereal
- 2 Tbsp. freshly grated parmesan cheese
- 1 ¼ tsp. smoked paprika
- ½ tsp. garlic powder
- ½ tsp. onion powder
- ¼ tsp. chili powder
- 1/8 tsp. black pepper

Method:

1. Set Air Crisp to 400 degrees and preheat for about 10 minutes. Spray the fryer basket lightly with cooking spray.
2. Season pork chops on both sides with kosher salt.
3. Combine panko bread crumbs, crushed cornflakes, parmesan cheese, ¾ tsp. kosher salt, paprika, garlic powder, onion powder, chili powder and black pepper in a large bowl.
4. Beat the egg in a smaller bowl. Dip the pork into the egg, then dredge in the crumb mixture.
5. When the Air Crisp basket is hot, place half of the porkchops into the basket.
6. Cook for 6 minutes, turn, and cook for 6 minutes more, lightly spraying the chops with oil spray after the turn. Remove the three porkchops and set aside, and repeat the process with the rest of the chops.

Nutrition Information Per Serving:

- Total Fat: 13 grams
- Carbohydrates: 8 grams
- Protein: 33 grams

Ninja Foodi Beef Meatballs

Servings: 4

Time Required: About 45 minutes

Ingredients:

- 1 ½ lb. ground beef (85 percent lean)
- 2 eggs
- ¾ cup Parmesan cheese, grated
- ¼ tsp. garlic powder
- ¼ tsp. onion powder
- ¼ tsp. oregano
- 1 tsp. kosher salt
- 2 Tbsp. chopped fresh parsley
- 3 cups sugar-free marinara sauce

Method:

1. In a medium mixing bowl, combine ground beef and seasonings by hand until thoroughly mixed.
2. Form into meatballs about 2 inches in diameter. You should get 12-15 meatballs.
3. Spray the pot lightly with olive oil spray.
4. Press the sauté button and brown the meatballs, turning to brown them on all sides.
5. Arrange the meatballs in the pot so that they are about a half inch apart. Pour sauce over meatballs.
6. Cover the pot and set to cook in the Pressure mode for 10 minutes.
7. After venting the pot carefully, remove the meatballs and sauce. Serve on their own or over cooked spaghetti squash.

Nutrition Information Per Serving (3 meatballs):

- Total Fat: 33 grams
- Carbohydrates: 5 grams
- Protein: 34 grams

Ninja Foodi Southwestern Chicken Wings

Servings: 4
Time Required: About 40 minutes
Ingredients:

- ½ cup water
- ½ cup prepared hot sauce
- 2 Tbsp. unsalted butter, melted
- 1 ½ Tbsp. apple cider vinegar
- 2 lb. frozen chicken wings
- 1 oz. prepared ranch salad dressing mix
- ½ tsp. paprika
- Olive oil cooking spray

Method:

1. Mix the water, hot pepper sauce, butter, and vinegar together in the pot. Add the wings to the Air Crisp basket, and put the basket in the pot. Close and lock the pot
2. Cook in Pressure mode at high pressure for 5 minutes.
3. When the cooking time is up, do a quick release of the pressure. When all pressure is released, carefully open the pot.
4. Sprinkle the chicken wings with the ranch dressing mix and paprika. Spray lightly with olive oil spray.
5. Set to Air Crisp at 375 degrees for 15 minutes.
6. Halfway through the crisping process, open the Foodi, stir the wings, and lightly spray them with oil again.
7. Remove after the wings are golden and crispy. Serve hot.

Nutrition Information Per Serving:

- Total Fat: 26 grams
- Carbohydrates: 1 gram
- Protein: 69 grams

Ninja Foodi Spicy Mocha Beef Roast

Servings: 8
Time Required: About an hour
Ingredients:

- 2 Tbsp. ground coffee
- 1 Tbsp. black pepper
- 1 Tbsp. cocoa powder
- 1 tsp. red chili flakes
- 1 tsp. chili powder
- 1 tsp. ground ginger
- 1 tsp. kosher salt
- 2 lb. beef chuck roast, cubed
- 2 cups beef stock
- 1 onion, chopped
- 3 Tbsp. balsamic vinegar
- Salt and pepper to taste

Method:

1. In a small bowl, combine ground coffee, black pepper, cocoa powder, chili flakes, chili powder, ginger and kosher salt.
2. In a medium bowl, toss cubed beef with the 3 tablespoons of the spice mixture until the meat is well coated.
3. Place the meat in the Ninja Foodi, and add the stock, onion and vinegar.
4. Press the Pressure button and set the cooking time for 35 minutes.
5. At the end of the cooking time, allow the pot to vent naturally.
6. When the pressure is fully released, remove the lid.
7. Serve the meat drizzled with the sauce from the pot.
8. Serves four.

Nutrition Information Per Serving:

- Total Fat: 10 grams
- Carbohydrates: 16 grams
- Protein: 48 grams

Ninja Foodi Lemon Garlic Chicken

Servings: 6
Time Required: About 35 minutes
Ingredients:

- 2 lb. chicken breasts or thighs
- 1 tsp. kosher salt
- 1 onion, chopped
- 1 Tbsp. olive oil
- 5 cloves garlic, minced
- ½ cup chicken stock

Method:

1. Press the sauté button on your pot and add the olive oil. When the oil is heated, after about a minute, add the onion. Sauté, stirring, until the onion is soft and translucent.
2. Add the chicken, stock, salt, and garlic. Cover and lock the pot.
3. Press the Pressure button and set cook time to 15 minutes.
4. At the end of the cook time, carefully vent the pot.
5. Remove the lid and serve chicken with sauce from the pot.
6. Serves four.

Nutrition Information Per Serving:

- Total Fat: 25 grams
- Carbohydrates: 9 grams
- Protein: 27 grams

Ninja Foodi Indian-Style Chicken

Servings: 3
Time Required: About an hour
Ingredients:

- 3 chicken breast fillets, boneless and skinless
- ½ onion, chopped
- ½ tsp. ground ginger
- 4 cloves garlic, minced
- 2 tsp. curry powder
- 2 tsp. ground cumin
- 1 Tbsp. cider vinegar
- 1 Tbsp. fresh lemon juice

Method:

1. Put all the ingredients in your Ninja Foodi's main pot. Cover and lock the pot.
2. Press the Pressure button and set the cook time to 40 minutes.
3. At the end of the cook time, carefully vent the pot manually.
4. Remove the chicken and shred.
5. Serve over roasted cauliflower. Serves three.

Nutrition Information Per Serving:

- Total Fat: 9 grams
- Carbohydrates: 3 grams
- Protein: 22 grams

Ninja Foodi Creamy Ranch Chicken

Servings: 4
Time Required: About 30 minutes
Ingredients:

- 1 head cauliflower, chopped
- 1 lb. chicken breast, boneless and skinless, cut into cubes
- ½ cup prepared ranch dressing
- 4 oz. cream cheese
- 2 cups shredded cheddar cheese
- Salt and pepper to taste

Method:

1. Add all the ingredients, excluding the cream cheese and cheddar cheese, to the Ninja Foodi.
2. Cover and lock the pot.
3. Using the Pressure mode, cook for 10 minutes.
4. At the end of the cooking time, allow the pot to vent naturally for 10 minutes. After 10 minutes, carefully vent any remaining steam and uncover the pot.
5. Stir in the cream cheese and cheddar cheese, continuing to stir until the cheese have melted.
6. Transfer to serving bowls and serve hot.

Nutrition Information Per Serving:

- Total Fat: 25 grams
- Carbohydrates: 8 grams
- Protein: 24 grams

Ninja Foodi Mediterranean Chicken

Servings: 6
Time Required: About an hour
Ingredients:

- 6 chicken thighs, with skin
- 2 Tbsp. olive oil
- 2 cloves garlic, crushed
- Salt and pepper
- ½ tsp. red chili flakes
- 14 oz. canned chopped tomatoes
- ½ cup black olives, pitted
- 1 Tbsp. capers
- 1 Tbsp. fresh basil, chopped
- ¾ cup water

Method:

1. Press the sauté button and add olive oil to the pot. Heat oil for a minute and then place chicken carefully in the pot, skin side down. Brown chicken without turning for about 5 minutes. When chicken is browned, remove from the pot and set aside.
2. Add tomatoes, olives, garlic, capers, basil, chili flakes and water to the pot. Season with salt and pepper to taste. Stir to combine and heat to a simmer.
3. When the mixture begins to simmer, add the chicken to the pot. Cover and lock the pot.
4. Using the Pressure mode, set the pot to cook for 15 minutes. At the end of the cooking time, allow pot to vent naturally for 10-15 minutes.
5. After 10-15 minutes, vent pot and remove chicken and sauce.
6. Serves six.

Nutrition Information Per Serving:

- Total Fat: 20 grams
- Carbohydrates: 10 grams
- Protein: 38 grams

Ninja Foodi Italian Chicken

Servings: 4
Time Required: About an hour
Ingredients:

- 4 chicken thighs, with the bone, skinless
- Salt and pepper to taste
- Olive oil spray
- 14 oz. crushed tomatoes
- ½ onion, diced
- 1 bell pepper, diced
- ½ tsp. oregano

Method:

1. Season chicken with salt and pepper, flipping to season both sides equally.
2. Press sauté on the Ninja Foodi and spray with a light coating of oil. Brown the chicken in the pot, turning to brown all sides, then remove from the pot and put aside.
3. Spray the pot with oil again, and then sauté onions and peppers until soft and beginning to brown, approximately 5 minutes.
4. Put the chicken back into the pot. Add tomatoes, oregano, bay leaf, salt and pepper. Stir and cover.
5. Cook in the Pressure mode for 25 minutes. Vent the pot carefully and remove chicken.
6. Serves four.

Nutrition Information Per Serving:

- Total Fat: 3 grams
- Carbohydrates: 10.5 grams
- Protein: 14 grams

Ninja Foodi Stroganoff

Servings: 4
Time Required: About 45 minutes
Ingredients:

- 1 Tbsp. olive oil
- ½ onion, chopped
- 1 clove garlic, minced
- 1 lb. beef stew meat
- 1 cup fresh mushrooms, chopped
- 1 Tbsp. Worcestershire sauce
- 1 tsp. salt
- ½ tsp. freshly ground black pepper
- ¾ cup water
- ½ cup sour cream

Method:

1. Press the Sauté button on the pot and add oil. When the oil is hot, add the onions to the pot and sauté until soft and translucent, about 5 minutes.
2. Add garlic to the pot and sauté for one minute more.
3. Add the beef to the pot and sauté until the meat is thoroughly browned on all sides, stirring constantly with a wooden spoon or spatula. This should take about 10 minutes.
4. Add the rest of the ingredients, excluding the sour cream, to the pot and stir to combine.
5. Cover and lock the pot and stop the Sauté cycle.
6. Using the Pressure mode, set the cook time to 15 minutes.
7. When the cooking time is finished allow the pot to vent naturally for 10 minutes.
8. After 10 minutes, carefully vent any remaining steam and remove lid.
9. Stir in the sour cream until it's thoroughly combined.
10. Serve hot over steamed cauliflower.

Nutrition Information Per Serving:

Total Fat: 16 grams
Carbohydrates: 9 grams
Protein: 33 grams

Ninja Foodi French-Style Beef Roast

Servings: 6
Time Required: About 1.25 hours
Ingredients:

- 3 lb. beef chuck roast
- 3 cloves garlic, minced
- 1 Tbsp. olive oil
- 1 tsp. salt
- ½ tsp. freshly ground black pepper
- ½ tsp. dried rosemary
- 1 Tbsp. butter
- ½ tsp. dried thyme
- ¼ cup balsamic vinegar
- 1 cup beef stock

Method:

1. In a small bowl, combine salt, pepper, rosemary and thyme. Rub the herb mixture on all sides of the roast.
2. Press the Sauté button on the pot and add oil. When the oil is hot, carefully place the roast into the pot and brown, turning it to evenly brown all sides.
3. Remove the roast from the pot and set aside.
4. Add the butter, vinegar, garlic and stock to the pot, stirring and scraping all the browned bits from the bottom of the pot.
5. Return the roast to the pot.
6. Cover and lock the pot and stop the Sauté cycle.
7. Using the Pressure mode, set the cook time to 40 minutes.
8. When the cooking time is finished allow the pot to vent naturally for 10 minutes.
9. After 10 minutes, carefully vent any remaining steam and remove lid.
10. Serve hot.

Nutrition Information Per Serving:

- Total Fat: 34 grams
- Carbohydrates: 3 grams
- Protein: 60 grams

Ninja Foodi Shepherd's Pie

Servings: 6
Time Required: About 45 minutes
Ingredients:

- 1 head cauliflower, core and leaves removed
- 4 Tbsp. butter
- 4 oz. cream cheese
- 1 egg
- 1 cup mozzarella cheese, grated
- Salt and pepper to taste
- 1 Tbsp. garlic powder
- 2 lb. ground beef, 90 percent lean
- 2 cups carrots, sliced
- 2 cups frozen peas
- 8 oz. fresh white mushrooms, sliced
- 1 cup beef stock

Method:

1. Put the steamer rack into the Ninja Foodi and pour in a cup of water. Place the cauliflower on the steamer rack. Cover and lock the pot.
2. Using the Pressure mode, cook for 5 minutes. Carefully vent the pot manually and uncover the pot.
3. Transfer cauliflower to a blender or food processor. Add the butter, cream cheese, mozzarella, egg, and salt and pepper. Blend until the mixture is smooth.
4. In a medium bowl, mix together the ground beef, carrots, peas and mushrooms.
5. Remove the steamer rack from the Ninja Foodi and drain any water.
6. Place the meat and vegetable mixture into the pot. Add the cauliflower mixture on top of the meat mixture.
7. Cover and lock the pot.
8. Using the Pressure mode, cook for 10 minutes.
9. At the end of the cooking time, manually vent the pot.
10. Spoon the hot shepherd's pie into serving bowls and serve immediately.

Nutrition Information Per Serving:

- Total Fat: 21 grams
- Carbohydrates: 4 grams
- Protein: 22 grams

Ninja Foodi Beef Brisket

Servings: 6
Time Required: About 1.25 hours
Ingredients:

- 2 lb. beef brisket
- ½ Tbsp. salt
- 2 tsp. freshly ground black pepper
- 2 onions, chopped
- ½ cup water
- 2 Tbsp. tomato paste
- 2 Tbsp. Worcestershire sauce

Method:

1. Place onions in the bottom of the Ninja Foodi's inner liner. Place the brisket on top of the onions.
2. In a small bowl, whisk together water, tomato paste and Worcestershire sauce. Pour the mixture over the brisket.
3. Cover and lock the pot.
4. Using the Pressure mode, cook for 60 minutes.
5. At the end of the cooking time, allow the pot to vent naturally for 10 minutes. After 10 minutes, carefully release any remaining steam and uncover the pot.
6. Transfer the brisket to a serving platter, topped with sauce from the pot.

Nutrition Information Per Serving:

- Total Fat: 8 grams
- Carbohydrates: 5 grams
- Protein: 24 grams

Ninja Foodi Chicken Vindaloo

Servings: 4
Time Required: About 10.5 hours
Ingredients:
- 1 lb. chicken thighs, boneless and skinless, cut into bite-size pieces
- 1 onion, diced
- 5 cloves garlic, minced
- 1 tsp. fresh ginger, peeled and minced
- 1 Tbsp. olive oil
- ¼ cup white vinegar
- 1 cup chopped tomato
- 1 tsp. salt
- 1 tsp. garam masala
- 1 tsp. smoked paprika
- ½ tsp. cayenne pepper
- ½ tsp. ground coriander
- ½ tsp. ground cumin
- ½ tsp. turmeric
- ¼ cup water

Method:
1. Press the Sauté button on the Ninja Foodi and heat the oil in it. Add the onions and sauté until they begin to brown, about 5 minutes. Add ginger and garlic and sauté for about a minute more.
2. Stop the Sauté cycle and transfer the onions, garlic and ginger, along with cayenne, coriander, cumin, salt and pepper, to a blender or food processor. Blend to a smooth consistency.
3. Transfer the mixture to a medium mixing bowl and add the chicken, tossing to coat. Add ¼ cup water and turmeric and mix well. Cover the bowl and allow to marinate in the refrigerator for up to 8 hours.
4. After marinating, transfer the mixture to the Ninja Foodi.
5. Using the Pressure mode, cook the chicken for 5 minutes.
6. At the end of the cooking time, allow the pot to vent naturally for 10 minutes. After 10 minutes, carefully vent any remaining steam and uncover the pot.
7. If you'd like the sauce to be thicker, press the Sauté button again and allow the sauce to reduce before serving.

Nutrition Information Per Serving:
- Total Fat: 8 grams
- Carbohydrates: 7 grams
- Protein: 23 grams

Ninja Foodi Chicken Tikka Masala

Servings: 6
Time Required: About 2.5 hours
Ingredients:

- 1 ½ lb. chicken breast, boneless and skinless, cut into bite-size pieces
- ½ cup Greek-style yogurt
- 9 cloves garlic, minced
- 4 tsp. fresh ginger, peeled and minced
- 1 ½ tsp. turmeric
- ¾ tsp. cayenne pepper
- 1 ½ tsp. smoked paprika
- 2 tsp. salt
- 3 tsp. garam masala
- 1 ½ tsp. ground cumin
- 1 onion, chopped
- 14 oz. canned diced tomatoes
- 1 carrot, chopped
- 4 oz. half and half
- 1 tsp. garam masala
- ½ cup chopped cilantro

Method:

1. In a medium bowl, mix together yogurt, 4 cloves garlic, 2 teaspoons ginger, ½ teaspoon turmeric, ¼ teaspoon cayenne, ½ teaspoon paprika, 1 teaspoon salt, 1 teaspoon garam masala and ½ teaspoon cumin.
2. Toss the chicken with this mixture and allow it to marinate for up to 2 hours.
3. Add onion, tomatoes, carrot, 5 cloves garlic, 2 teaspoons ginger, 1 teaspoon turmeric, ½ teaspoon cayenne, 1 teaspoon paprika, 1 teaspoon salt, 2 teaspoons garam masala and 1 teaspoon cumin to the Ninja Foodi.
4. Add marinated chicken to the pot, too.
5. Using the Pressure mode, cook for 10 minutes.
6. At the end of the cooking time, carefully vent the pot manually.
7. Remove the chicken from the sauce and set aside.
8. If you have an immersion blender, use it to puree the sauce in the pot. Otherwise, transfer the sauce to a blender or food processor and blend until smooth.
9. Stir in the half and half.
10. Return the chicken to the sauce and serve hot, garnished with cilantro.

Nutrition Information Per Serving:

- Total Fat: 6 grams
- Carbohydrates: 10 grams
- Protein: 18 grams

Ninja Foodi Asian Spareribs

Servings: 2
Time Required: About 45 minutes
Ingredients:

- 1 ½ lb. pork spareribs, cut into serving-size pieces
- 1 Tbsp. olive oil
- 1 clove garlic, minced
- 1 Tbsp. fresh ginger, peeled and minced
- 2 Tbsp. black bean sauce
- 1 Tbsp. wine vinegar
- 1 Tbsp. soy sauce
- 1 Tbsp. honey
- ¼ cup water
- ½ cup spring onions, chopped

Method:

1. Press the Sauté button on the pot and add oil. When the oil is hot, sauté the garlic and ginger just until fragrant, about 30 seconds.
2. Add bean sauce, vinegar, soy sauce, honey and water to the pot, stirring to combine.
3. Add ribs to the pot and turn to coat them with the sauce.
4. Cover and lock the pot.
5. Using the Pressure mode, set the cook time to 15 minutes.
6. At the end of the cook time, allow the pot to vent naturally for 10 minutes.
7. After 10 minutes, carefully vent any remaining steam and remove the cover.
8. Remove the ribs with tongs or a slotted spoon and serve garnished with chopped spring onions.

Nutrition Information Per Serving:

Total Fat: 32 grams

Carbohydrates: 5 grams

Protein: 19 grams

Ninja Foodi Leg of Lamb

Servings: 4
Time Required: About 1.5 hours
Ingredients:

- 1 lb. leg of lamb, cubed
- 1 cup onion, diced
- 4 cloves garlic, minced
- 2 tsp. fresh ginger, peeled and minced
- 2 tsp. garam masala
- 1 tsp. smoked paprika
- 1 tsp. salt
- 1 tsp. turmeric
- ½ tsp. ground cinnamon
- ¼ tsp. cayenne pepper
- ¼ cup yogurt
- 1 Tbsp. tomato paste
- ¼ cup fresh cilantro, chopped

Method:

1. Combine all ingredients in a mixing bowl, stirring until lamb is thoroughly coated with the yogurt-spice mixture.
2. Cover the bowl with plastic wrap and refrigerate for at least an hour.
3. After the meat has had a chance to marinate, transfer everything to the Ninja Foodi.
4. Cover and lock the pot.
5. Using the Pressure mode, set a cook time of 20 minutes.
6. At the end of the cooking time, allow the pot to vent naturally for 10 minutes.
7. After 10 minutes, carefully vent any remaining steam and remove the cover.
8. Serve the meat hot alone or over steamed cauliflower.

Nutrition Information Per Serving:

- Total Fat: 3 grams
- Carbohydrates: 6 grams
- Protein: 16 grams

Ninja Foodi Ham and Greens

Servings: 6
Time Required: About 20 minutes
Ingredients:

- 6 cups collard greens, chopped
- 2 cups cooked ham, diced
- 1 onion, diced
- 6 cloves garlic, minced
- 1 tsp. salt
- 1 tsp. freshly ground black pepper
- ¼ cup water
- ½ tsp. red pepper flakes
- 1 tsp. dried thyme
- 1 Tbsp. cider vinegar
- 1 tsp. red chili hot sauce

Method:

1. Place all ingredients except vinegar and hot sauce in the Ninja Foodi.
2. Cover and lock the pot.
3. Using the Pressure mode, set the cook time for 4 minutes.
4. At the end of the cooking time, allow the pot to vent naturally for 5 minutes.
5. After five minutes, carefully vent any remaining steam and remove the cover.
6. Stir in vinegar and hot sauce.
7. Serve hot.

Nutrition Information Per Serving:

- Total Fat: 2 grams
- Carbohydrates: 9 grams
- Protein: 4 grams

Ninja Foodi Mushroom Pork Chops

Servings: 4
Time Required: About an hour
Ingredients:

- 4 pork loin chops, boneless
- 1 Tbsp. paprika
- 1 tsp. garlic powder
- 1 tsp. onion powder
- 1 tsp. freshly ground black pepper
- 1 tsp. salt
- ¼ tsp. cayenne pepper
- 1 Tbsp. olive oil
- ½ onion, chopped
- 6 oz. button mushrooms, sliced
- 1 Tbsp. butter
- ½ cup heavy cream

Method:

1. In a small bowl, combine paprika, garlic powder, onion powder, black pepper, salt and cayenne pepper.
2. Rub both sides of the pork chops with 1 tablespoon of the spice mixture.
3. Press the Sauté button on the pot and add oil. When the oil is hot, sauté the pork chops to brown them on both sides, about 3 minutes per side. Remove the chops from the pot and set aside.
4. Stop the Sauté cycle.
5. Add the onions and mushrooms to the pot.
6. Place the pork chops back into the pot on top of the onions and mushrooms.
7. Cover and lock the pot.
8. Using the Pressure mode, set the cook time for 25 minutes and start the cook cycle.
9. At the end of the cooking time, carefully vent the pot manually.
10. Remove the cover and transfer the pork chops to a serving platter.
11. Press the Sauté button on the Ninja Foodi.
12. Stir in butter and cream and heat, stirring, for about 5 minutes until the butter is melted.
13. Drizzle the sauce over the pork chops and serve.

Nutrition Information Per Serving:

- Total Fat: 32 grams
- Carbohydrates: 7 grams
- Protein: 40 grams

Ninja Foodi Mexican Chicken

Servings: 6
Time Required: About 45 minutes
Ingredients:

- 2 lb. boneless skinless chicken thighs boneless, chopped
- 1 Tbsp. ground cumin
- 1 Tbsp. chili powder
- 1 Tbsp. salt
- 2 Tbsp. olive oil
- 14 oz. canned diced tomatoes
- 5 oz. tomato paste
- 1 onion, chopped
- 3 cloves garlic, minced

Method:

1. In a medium bowl, combine cumin, chili powder and salt. Toss the chicken in the spice mixture to coat.
2. Press the Sauté button on the Ninja Foodi and heat the oil. When the oil is hot, sauté the chicken for about 5 minutes.
3. Stop the Sauté cycle and then add all the other ingredients to the pot.
4. Cover and lock the pot.
5. Using the Pressure mode, cook for 15 minutes.
6. At the end of the cooking time, allow the pot to vent naturally for 10 minutes. After 10 minutes, carefully vent any remaining pressure and uncover the pot.
7. Transfer for to a serving platter and serve hot.

Nutrition Information Per Serving:

- Total Fat: 22 grams
- Carbohydrates: 4 grams
- Protein: 19 grams

Ninja Foodi Chicken Korma

Servings: 4
Time Required: About 45 minutes
Ingredients:

- 1 lb. chicken thighs, boneless and skinless, cut into bite-size pieces
- 1 oz. unsalted cashews
- 1 onion, chopped
- ½ cup tomatoes, diced
- ½ Serrano chili pepper, seeded and chopped
- 5 cloves garlic, minced
- 1 tsp. fresh ginger, peeled and minced
- 1 tsp. turmeric
- 1 tsp. salt
- 1 tsp. garam masala
- ½ tsp. cumin
- ½ tsp. coriander
- ½ tsp. cayenne pepper
- ½ cup water
- ½ cup unsweetened coconut milk

Method:

1. In a blender or food processor, combine cashews, onion, tomatoes, chili pepper, ginger, garlic, turmeric, salt, garam masala, cumin, coriander and cayenne. Blend until the mixture is smooth.
2. Pour the blended mixture into the Ninja Foodi. Use ½ cup water to rinse the blender jar, and pour the water into the pot.
3. Stir the chicken into the mixture in the pot.
4. Cover and lock the pot.
5. Using the Pressure mode, cook for 10 minutes.
6. When the cooking time is done, allow the pot to vent naturally for 10 minutes. After 10 minutes, carefully vent any remaining pressure and uncover the pot.
7. Stir in the coconut milk and serve the mixture hot, garnished with chopped fresh cilantro.

Nutrition Information Per Serving:

- Total Fat: 19 grams
- Carbohydrates: 6 grams
- Protein: 14 grams

Ninja Foodi Butter Chicken

Servings: 8
Time Required: About 35 minutes
Ingredients:

- 2 lb. chicken thighs, boneless and skinless, cut into large pieces
- 14 oz. canned diced tomatoes
- 6 cloves garlic, minced
- 2 tsp. fresh ginger, peeled and minced
- 1 tsp. turmeric
- ½ tsp. cayenne pepper
- 1 tsp. paprika
- 1 tsp. salt
- 1 tsp. garam masala
- 1 tsp. ground cumin
- 4 oz. butter, cubed
- 4 oz. heavy cream

Method:

1. Put tomatoes, garlic, ginger, turmeric, cayenne, paprika, salt, garam masala, and cumin in the Ninja Foodi. Mix well.
2. Add the chicken to the pot, tossing to coat it with the sauce ingredients.
3. Cover and lock the pot.
4. Using the Pressure mode, cook at high pressure.
5. At the end of the cooking time, allow the pot to vent naturally for 10 minutes. After 10 minutes, carefully release any remaining pressure and uncover the pot.
6. Transfer the chicken to a plate and set aside.
7. Using an immersion blender, blend the sauce until it's smooth.
8. Add the butter and cream, stirring until the butter is melted.
9. Return the chicken to the pot and mix well.
10. Transfer to a serving platter and serve hot, garnished with chopped fresh cilantro.

Nutrition Information Per Serving:

- Total Fat: 20 grams
- Carbohydrates: 3 grams
- Protein: 25 grams

Ninja Foodi Garlic Chicken

Servings: 4
Time Required: About 1.25 hours
Ingredients:

- 1 lb. chicken thighs, boneless and skinless
- 2 tsp. Herbs de Provence
- 1 Tbsp. olive oil
- 1 Tbsp. Dijon mustard
- 1 Tbsp. cider vinegar
- 1 tsp. salt
- 1 tsp. freshly ground black pepper
- 2 cloves garlic, minced
- 2 Tbsp. butter
- 8 cloves garlic, sliced
- ¼ cup water
- ¼ cup heavy cream

Method:

1. In a medium bowl, mix together herbs, olive oil, mustard, vinegar, minced garlic, salt and pepper. Toss the chicken in the mixture to coat. Cover with plastic wrap and allow to marinate at room temperature for 30 minutes.
2. Press the Sauté button on the Ninja Foodi and heat the butter in the pot. When the butter has melted, add the sliced garlic and sauté just until the garlic is fragrant, about a minute.
3. Add the chicken to the pot, reserving the marinade in the bowl. Sauté the chicken to brown it on both sides, turning it halfway through. This should take about 2 minutes per side.
4. Add the marinade to the pot, along with about ¼ cup water.
5. Cover the pot and continue to sauté for about 10 minutes, turning the chicken once during the process. Your goal is to get the chicken to an internal temperature of 165 degrees Fahrenheit; you can use a meat thermometer to check.
6. When the chicken has reached the correct temperature, transfer it to a serving platter.
7. Stir the cream into the pot and heat the sauce thoroughly.
8. When the sauce has thickened slightly, pour it over the chicken and serve immediately.

Nutrition Information Per Serving:

- Total Fat: 37 grams
- Carbohydrates: 4 grams
- Protein: 19 grams

Ninja Foodi Beef Curry

Servings: 6
Time Required: About an hour
Ingredients:

- 1 ½ lb. beef stew meat
- 1 onion, chopped
- 2 tomatoes, chopped
- 4 cloves garlic
- ½ cup fresh cilantro, chopped
- 1 tsp. cumin
- ½ tsp. coriander
- 1 tsp. garam masala
- ½ tsp. cayenne pepper
- Salt to taste

Method:

1. In a blender or food processor, blend the onion, tomatoes, garlic, cilantro, cumin, coriander, garam masala, cayenne, and salt to a smooth puree.
2. Put the meat into the Ninja Foodi, and then pour the vegetable puree over the top of the meat.
3. Cover and lock the pot.
4. Using the Pressure mode, cook for 30 minutes.
5. At the end of the cooking time, allow the pot to vent naturally for 10 minutes. After 10 minutes, carefully release any remaining steam and uncover the pot.
6. Serve the curry hot over riced cauliflower, garnished with chopped fresh cilantro.

Nutrition Information Per Serving:

- Total Fat: 8 grams
- Carbohydrates: 4 grams
- Protein: 31 grams

Ninja Foodi Shawarma

Servings: 4
Time Required: About 30 minutes
Ingredients:

- 2 tsp. dried oregano
- 1 tsp. ground cinnamon
- ½ tsp. ground allspice
- ½ tsp. cayenne pepper
- 1 tsp. ground cumin
- 1 tsp. ground coriander
- 1 tsp. salt
- 1 lb. ground beef, 90 percent lean
- 1 onion, sliced
- 1 red bell pepper, chopped
- 2 cups cabbage, chopped

Method:

1. In a small bowl, mix oregano, cinnamon, allspice, cayenne, cumin, coriander, and salt.
2. Press the Sauté button on your Ninja Foodi, and when the pot is hot, add the ground beef. Sauté, stirring, until the meat is thoroughly browned.
3. When the meat is well browned, add 2 tablespoons of the spice mixture and stir to combine.
4. Add the onions, bell pepper and cabbage.
5. Stop the Sauté cycle and cover and lock the pot.
6. Using the Pressure mode, cook for 2 minutes.
7. At the end of the cooking time, allow the pot to vent naturally for 5 minutes. After 5 minutes, carefully release any remaining pressure and uncover the pot.
8. Serve the shawarma hot.

Nutrition Information Per Serving:

- Total Fat: 5 grams
- Carbohydrates: 8 grams
- Protein: 25 grams

Ninja Foodi Beef Stew

Servings: 4
Time Required: About 30 minutes
Ingredients:

- 1 lb. ground beef, 90 percent lean
- 5 oz. canned tomato sauce
- 2 Tbsp. tomato paste
- 2 cups frozen sweet corn
- 1 cup frozen carrots
- 3 Tbsp. cider vinegar
- 1 Tbsp. soy sauce
- 1 tsp. salt
- 2 tsp. freshly ground black pepper

Method:

1. Press the Sauté button on your Ninja Foodi, and when the pot is hot, add the ground beef. Sauté, stirring, until the meat is thoroughly browned.
2. When the meat is well browned, add the rest of the ingredients and stop the Sauté cycle.
3. Cover and lock the pot.
4. Using the Pressure mode, cook for 5 minutes.
5. At the end of the cooking time, allow the pot to vent naturally for 10 minutes. After 10 minutes, carefully release any remaining pressure and uncover the pot.
6. Serve the stew hot, garnished with chopped fresh parsley.

Nutrition Information Per Serving:

- Total Fat: 4 grams
- Carbohydrates: 20 grams
- Protein: 19 grams

Ninja Foodi Barbecue Ribs

Servings: 4
Time Required: About 45 minutes
Ingredients:

- 1 tsp. dried oregano
- 1 tsp. garlic powder
- 1 tsp. onion powder
- ½ tsp. smoked paprika
- ½ tsp. dry mustard
- ¼ tsp. cayenne powder
- ½ tsp. salt
- ¼ tsp. freshly ground black pepper
- 2 lb. pork baby back ribs, cut into serving-size pieces
- 1 cup water
- ½ cup cider vinegar

Method:

1. In a small bowl, mix oregano, garlic powder, onion powder, paprika, mustard, cayenne, salt and pepper.
2. Rub the ribs thoroughly on all sides with the spice mixture.
3. Place the steamer rack in your Ninja Foodi. Pour in the water and vinegar.
4. Place the ribs on the steamer rack.
5. Cover and lock the pot.
6. Using the Pressure mode, cook for 20 minutes.
7. After the cooking cycle has ended, allow the pot to vent naturally for 10 minutes. After 10 minutes, carefully vent any remaining steam and uncover the pot.
8. Place the ribs under a hot broiler to brown them, about 2 minutes per side.

Nutrition Information Per Serving:

- Total Fat: 40 grams
- Carbohydrates: 1 gram
- Protein: 65 grams

Ninja Foodi Spicy Chicken

Servings: 6
Time Required: About an hour
Ingredients:

- 1 ½ lb. chicken thighs, boneless and skinless
- 1 Tbsp. olive oil
- 2 tomatillos, thinly sliced
- ½ onion, thinly sliced
- 4 cloves garlic, minced
- 1/3 cup chicken stock
- 7 oz. canned roasted tomatoes
- 1 Tbsp. adobo chipotle chili, chopped
- ½ tsp. ground cumin
- ¼ tsp. ground cinnamon
- ½ tsp. dried oregano
- 1 Tbsp. soy sauce
- 1 Tbsp. cider vinegar

Method:

1. Press the Sauté button on the Ninja Foodi and heat the oil in the pot. When the oil is hot, add the tomatillos and onions. Sauté until the vegetables are browned, about 7-10 minutes.
2. Add the garlic and sauté a minute more.
3. Add chicken stock and tomatoes, stirring to deglaze the pot liner.
4. Add the chipotle chili, cumin, cinnamon, oregano, soy sauce, and vinegar. Sauté until fragrant, about another minute.
5. Add the chicken and stop the Sauté cycle.
6. Cover and lock the pot.
7. Using the Chicken/Meat mode, cook for 15 minutes.
8. At the end of the cook time, allow the pot to vent naturally for 10 minutes, After 10 minutes, carefully release any remaining pressure and uncover the pot.
9. Remove the chicken and transfer to a plate. Allow it to cool slightly and then shred it with a fork or your fingers.
10. Using an immersion blender, blend the sauce in the Ninja Foodi until it's a smooth puree.
11. Press the Sauté button again and return the chicken to pot. Allow the pot to reheat until the mixture is heated through and the sauce has thickened a bit.
12. Serve the chicken with its sauce over riced cauliflower.

Nutrition Information Per Serving:

- Total Fat: 7 grams
- Carbohydrates: 4 grams
- Protein: 25 grams

Ninja Foodi Carne Adovada

Servings: 8
Time Required: About 45 minutes
Ingredients:

- 2 lb. pork shoulder, cut into bite-size pieces
- ¼ cup soy sauce
- 1 tsp. olive oil
- 1 onion, chopped
- 3 cloves garlic, minced
- 1 tsp. salt
- 1 tsp. oregano
- 1 Tbsp. cider vinegar
- 1 can chipotle chiles in adobo sauce
- ¼ cup chili powder

Method:

1. In a blender or food processor, combine onion, garlic, salt, oregano, chipotles, vinegar, soy sauce, and chili powder. Blend until the mixture is a smooth puree.
2. Put the pork into the Ninja Foodi. Pour the seasoning mixture over the pork. Use ¼ cup water to rinse the blender jar, and add the water to the pot, too.
3. Cover and lock the pot.
4. Using the Pressure mode, cook for 20 minutes.
5. At the end of the cooking time, carefully vent the pot manually.
6. Uncover the pot and transfer the meat with its sauce to a serving platter and serve hot.

Nutrition Information Per Serving

- Total Fat: 5 grams
- Carbohydrates: 5 grams
- Protein: 14 grams

Ninja Foodi Low-Carb Lasagna

Servings: 4
Time Required: About an hour
Ingredients:

- 1 lb. ground beef, 90 percent lean
- 2 cloves garlic, minced
- 1 onion, chopped
- 1 ½ cups ricotta cheese
- ½ cup Parmesan cheese
- 1 egg
- 25 oz. jarred marinara sauce
- 8 oz. mozzarella cheese, sliced

Method:

1. In a small bowl, stir the parmesan cheese into the ricotta cheese until well combined.
2. Press the Sauté button on the Ninja Foodi and allow the pot to heat. When the pot is hot, add the ground beef and brown the meat, stirring to break it up as it browns. This should take about 10 minutes.
3. When the meat is browned, add the onions and sauté for 5-7 minutes more. Add the garlic and sauté for one more minute.
4. Carefully drain excess grease from the meat mixture. Stir the marinara sauce into the meat mixture and transfer half of it to a baking dish that's small enough to fit into your Ninja Foodi.
5. Lay a third of the mozzarella slices on top of the meat sauce in the dish, and then spread half the ricotta mixture on top of the mozzarella.
6. Repeat the process in a second layer, putting the rest of the meat sauce on top of the ricotta, followed by another third of the mozzarella slices and the other half of the ricotta mixture.
7. Finish the layering by putting the remaining mozzarella slices on top of everything in the dish.
8. Cover the dish with aluminum foil.
9. Put the steamer rack in the Ninja Foodi and pour in a cup of water.
10. Place the covered baking dish on the steamer rack. Cover and lock the pot.
11. Using the Pressure mode, cook for 10 minutes.
12. At the end of the cooking time, carefully vent the pot manually and uncover the pot.
13. Allow the lasagna to cool for a few minutes and then spoon into serving bowls.

Nutrition Information Per Serving:

- Total Fat: 25 grams
- Carbohydrates: 7 grams
- Protein: 25 grams

Ninja Foodi Cheesy Bacon Ranch Chicken

Servings: 8

Time Required: About 30 minutes

Ingredients:

- 8 slices bacon, cooked crisp and crumbled
- 2 lb. chicken breast, boneless and skinless, cut into large pieces
- 1 packet ranch dressing mix
- 8 oz. cream cheese
- ½ cup water
- 1 cup cheddar cheese, grated

Method:

1. Place the chicken, cream cheese and water into the Ninja Foodi.
2. Sprinkle the ranch dressing mix over the top of the chicken and cream cheese.
3. Cover and lock the pot.
4. Using the Pressure mode, cook for 15 minutes.
5. At the end of the cooking time, carefully vent the pot manually.
6. Uncover the pot.
7. Press the Sauté button on the Ninja Foodi.
8. Stir in the bacon and cheddar cheese, continuing to stir as the mixture reheats until the cheese is melted.
9. Stop the Sauté cycle and transfer to serving bowls. Serve hot.

Nutrition Information Per Serving:

- Total Fat: 34 grams
- Carbohydrates: 2 grams
- Protein: 58 grams

Fish and Seafood

Seafood is an excellent source of protein and healthy fatty acids. Every diet should include them. Use these recipes to get fish and seafood onto your weekly menu in a way you'll love, and with unbelievable speediness, thanks to the Ninja Foodi.

Ninja Foodi Crispy Catfish

Servings: 4
Time Required: About 25 minutes
Ingredients:

- 4 catfish fillets, 6 oz. each
- ½ cup fine bread crumbs
- Olive oil cooking spray

Method:

1. Lightly spray each fish fillet with olive oil spray, then roll the fillets in bread crumbs. Season with salt and pepper, then give the fillets another spritz of oil.
2. Place the fillets in the Air Crisp basket, then put the basket in the Foodi pot.
3. Set to Air Crisp at 390 degrees for 10 minutes.
4. Open the Foodi, flip the fish, and spritz again with oil.
5. Close the pot and cook for another 10 minutes.

Nutrition Information Per Serving:

- Total Fat: 2 grams
- Carbohydrates: 0 gram
- Protein: 15 grams

Ninja Foodi Jambalaya

Servings: 6
Time Required: About 40 minutes
Ingredients:

- 1 lb. cooked, peeled shrimp
- 1 lb. cooked chicken breast, cubed
- 1 lb. andouille sausage, sliced
- ½ cup chicken stock
- ½ onion, diced
- 1 bell pepper, diced
- 14 oz. crushed tomato
- 2 cloves garlic, minced
- 1 Tbsp. olive oil
- 1 Tbsp. Cajun seasoning
- ½ tsp. hot sauce

Method:

1. Press the sauté button and add the olive oil. When the oil is hot, add the onion and bell pepper and sauté until soft. Add the garlic and sauté 1 minute more.
2. Add the sausage to the pot and sauté, stirring, until the sausage is brown.
3. Add the rest of the ingredients, then cover and lock the pot.
4. Using the Pressure function, set the cook time for 10 minutes.
5. At the end of the cook time, allow the pot to vent naturally, releasing any remaining pressure after 10 minutes.
6. Serve the jambalaya over steamed cauliflower.

Nutrition Information Per Serving:

- Total Fat: 9 grams
- Carbohydrates: 15 grams
- Protein: 32 grams

Ninja Foodi Fish Curry

Servings: 2
Time Required: About 35 minutes
Ingredients:

- 1 lb. firm fish such as halibut or cod
- 1 onion, chopped
- 3 cloves garlic, minced
- 2 Tbsp. fresh ginger, peeled and minced
- 1 tomato, chopped
- ¼ cup unsweetened coconut, shredded
- 3 tsp. olive oil
- 2 tsp. turmeric
- ¼ tsp. dry mustard
- ¼ tsp. cumin
- ¼ tsp. cayenne pepper
- 1 tsp. garam masala
- 1 cup water
- Salt to taste

Method:

1. Press the Sauté button on the pot and add oil. When the oil is hot, add the onions to the pot and sauté until soft and translucent, about 5 minutes.
2. Add garlic to the pot and sauté for one minute more.
3. Stir in tomato, spices, coconut and water. Cook until the sauce has thickened, about 5 minutes.
4. Add the fish to the pot and stir to combine.
5. Cover and lock the pot and stop the Sauté cycle.
6. Using the Pressure function, set the cook time for 10 minutes.
7. At the end of the cook time, allow the pot to vent naturally, releasing any remaining pressure after 10 minutes.
8. Serve the fish and sauce over cauliflower.

Nutrition Information Per Serving:

- Total Fat: 8 grams
- Carbohydrates: 7 grams
- Protein: 24 grams

Ninja Foodi Asian Salmon

Servings: 2
Time Required: About 45 minutes
Ingredients:

- 1 lb. salmon filets
- 1 Tbsp. soy sauce
- 2 tsp. fresh ginger, peeled and minced
- 1 clove garlic, minced
- ½ tsp. salt
- 1 tsp. freshly ground black pepper

Method:

1. In a small bowl, mix soy sauce, garlic, ginger, salt and pepper.
2. Place salmon in a pan that's small enough to fit into your Ninja Foodi.
3. Pour seasoning mixture over the salmon. Allow the fish to marinate for 30 minutes.
4. Place the steamer rack in the Ninja Foodi and pour 2 cups water into the pot.
5. Place the pan with the salmon onto the steamer rack.
6. Cover and lock the pot.
7. Using the Pressure function, set the cook time for 3 minutes.
8. At the end of the cook time, allow the pot to vent naturally for 5 minutes.
9. After 5 minutes, carefully vent any remaining steam and uncover the pot.
10. Transfer the salmon to serving plates and serve hot.

Nutrition Information Per Serving

- Total Fat: 7 grams
- Carbohydrates: 0 gram
- Protein: 23 grams

Ninja Foodi Ginger Garlic Fish

Servings: 2

Time Required: About 45 minutes

Ingredients:

- 1 lb. firm fish, such as tilapia or flounder
- 3 Tbsp. soy sauce
- 2 Tbsp. rice wine
- 1 Tbsp. black bean paste
- 1 tsp. fresh ginger, peeled and minced
- 1 clove garlic, minced

Method:

1. In a small bowl, mix together soy sauce, rice wine, bean paste, ginger and garlic. Season with salt and pepper.
2. Pour the seasoning mixture over the fish and allow to marinate for 30 minutes.
3. Place the steamer rack in the Ninja Foodi and pour in 2 cups of water.
4. Place the fish in a steamer basket, and place the basket on top of the steamer rack.
5. Cover and lock the pot.
6. Using the Pressure mode, cook for 2 minutes.
7. At the end of the cooking time, manually vent the pot immediately.
8. Uncover the pot and remove the basket.
9. Serve the fish hot, garnished with chopped spring onions.

Nutrition Information Per Serving:

- Total Fat: 3 grams
- Carbohydrates: 4 grams
- Protein: 24 grams

Ninja Foodi Spicy Cod

Servings: 2
Time Required: About 25 minutes
Ingredients:

- 1 lb. cod filets
- 1 onion, chopped
- 1 bell pepper, chopped
- 1 jalapeno pepper, seeded and chopped
- 2 small tomatoes, chopped
- 2 cloves garlic, minced
- 2 cups chicken stock
- 1 tsp. kosher salt
- ¼ tsp. black pepper
- 1 Tbsp. olive oil

Method:

1. Press the sauté button and add the olive oil. When the oil is hot, add the onions, jalapeno, and bell pepper and sauté until soft. Add the garlic and sauté 1 minute more.
2. Add the rest of the ingredients, then cover and lock the pot.
3. Using the Pressure function, set the cook time for 10 minutes.
4. At the end of the cook time, allow the pot to vent naturally, releasing any remaining pressure after 10 minutes.
5. Serve the fish and sauce over cauliflower.

Nutrition Information Per Serving:

- Total Fat: 5 grams
- Carbohydrates: 9.5 grams
- Protein: 11 grams

Ninja Foodi Coconut Shrimp

Servings: 3
Time Required: About 15 minutes
Ingredients:

- 1 lb. shrimp, peeled and uncooked
- 1 Tbsp. fresh ginger, peeled and minced
- 3 cloves garlic, minced
- ½ tsp. turmeric
- 1 tsp. salt
- ½ tsp. cayenne pepper
- 1 tsp. garam masala
- 8 oz. unsweetened coconut milk

Method:

1. In a mixing bowl, combine all ingredients, tossing in shrimp to thoroughly coat them with the seasoning mixture.
2. Transfer mixture to a pan that's small enough to fit in your Ninja Foodi. Cover the pan with foil.
3. Place the steamer rack in the Ninja Foodi and pour in 2 cups of water.
4. Place the pan with the shrimp onto the steamer rack.
5. Using the Pressure mode, set the cook time for 4 minutes.
6. At the end of the cook time, carefully vent the pot manually.
7. Serve hot.

Nutrition Information Per Serving:

- Total Fat: 12 grams
- Carbohydrates: 4 grams
- Protein: 16 grams

Ninja Foodi Greek Shrimp

Servings: 3
Time Required: About 15 minutes
Ingredients:

- 1 lb. shrimp, peeled
- 2 Tbsp. butter
- 3 cloves garlic, minced
- ½ tsp. red pepper flakes
- 1 onion, chopped
- 14 oz. canned diced tomatoes
- 1 tsp. dried oregano
- 1 tsp. salt
- 1 cup feta cheese, crumbled
- ½ cup black olives, sliced
- ¼ cup fresh parsley, chopped

Method:

1. Press the Sauté button on the Ninja Foodi and heat the butter in the pot. Once the butter has melted, add the onion and pepper flakes and sauté until the onion is translucent, about 5 minutes. Add the garlic and sauté for about a minute more.
2. Stop the Sauté cycle.
3. Add the tomatoes, oregano, salt and shrimp.
4. Cover and lock the pot.
5. Using the Pressure mode, cook for 1 minute.
6. After the end of the cooking time, carefully vent the pot quickly and remove the cover.
7. Transfer to a serving platter and top with feta, olives and parsley.
8. Serve with riced cauliflower.

Nutrition Information Per Serving:

Total Fat: 11 grams

Carbohydrates: 6 grams

Protein: 19 grams

Basic Ninja Foodi Shrimp

Servings: 6
Time Required: About 15 minutes
Ingredients:

- 2 lb. shrimp, peeled and cooked
- 2 Tbsp. olive oil
- 2 Tbsp. butter
- 2 cloves garlic, minced
- ½ cup white wine
- ½ cup chicken stock

Method:

1. Press the sauté button and add the olive oil. Add the garlic and sauté 1 minute.
2. Add the rest of the ingredients, then cover and lock the pot.
3. Using the Pressure function, set the cook time for 1 minute.
4. At the end of the cook time, allow the pot to vent naturally, releasing any remaining pressure after 5 minutes.
5. Serve the shrimp over steamed cauliflower.

Nutrition Information Per Serving:

- Total Fat: 4 grams
- Carbohydrates: 1 gram
- Protein: 21 grams

Ninja Foodi Lobster

Servings: 2

Time Required: About 15 minutes

Ingredients:

- 2 lb. live lobster
- 1 cup white wine
- 3 cups water

Method:

1. Add the water and wine to the pot.
2. Put the live lobster in the pot, then cover and lock the pot.
3. Using the Pressure function, set the cook time for 3 minutes.
4. At the end of the cook time, carefully vent the pot manually.
5. Allow the lobster to cool slightly before serving.

Nutrition Information Per Serving:

- Total Fat: 1 gram
- Carbohydrates: 2 grams
- Protein: 36 grams

Ninja Foodi Crab Legs

Servings: 2
Time Required: About 15 minutes
Ingredients:

- 2 lb. frozen crab legs
- ¾ cups water
- Butter

Method:

1. Fresh lemons, quartered
2. Place steamer basket in the pot.
3. Add the water to the pot.
4. Put the crab legs into the pot, then cover and lock the pot.
5. Using the Pressure function, set the cook time for 2 minutes.
6. At the end of the cook time, carefully vent the pot manually.
7. Serve the crab legs hot with melted butter and lemon quarters.

Nutrition Information Per Serving (excluding butter):

- Total Fat: 1 gram
- Carbohydrates: 0 gram
- Protein: 38 grams

Ninja Foodi Crab and Eggs

Servings: 2
Time Required: About 1.25 hours
Ingredients:

- 4 eggs, beaten
- 8 oz. lump crab meat or imitation crab
- 1 cup half and half
- ½ tsp. salt
- 1 tsp. freshly ground pepper
- 1 tsp. smoked paprika
- ½ tsp. dried thyme
- 1 cup Swiss cheese, grated
- 1 cup spring onions, chopped

Method:

1. In a mixing bowl, whisk together eggs and half and half.
2. Whisk in salt, pepper, thyme, and paprika.
3. Stir in cheese and spring onions.
4. Stir in crab meat.
5. Pour mixture into a pan that's small enough to fit into your Ninja Foodi. Cover the pan with foil.
6. Place steamer rack in the Ninja Foodi. Pour 2 cups water into the pot.
7. Place pan on rack in the Ninja Foodi.
8. Using the Pressure setting, set the cook time for 40 minutes.
9. At the end of the cook time, allow the pot to vent naturally for 10 minutes.
10. After 10 minutes, carefully release any remaining steam and remove the cover.
11. Serve the crab bake hot or allow to cool to room temperature.

Nutrition Information Per Serving:

- Total Fat: 25 grams
- Carbohydrates: 19 grams
- Protein: 22 grams

Ninja Foodi Teriyaki Scallops

Servings: 2
Time Required: About 15 minutes
Ingredients:

- 1 Tbsp. olive oil
- 1 lb. fresh sea scallops
- ½ cup coconut-based soy-style sauce
- 3 Tbsp. 100% maple syrup
- ½ tsp. garlic powder
- ½ tsp. ground ginger
- ½ tsp. kosher salt

Method:

1. Press the sauté button and heat the olive oil in the pot.
2. When the oil is hot, add the scallops and sear, turning so that they brown on both sides, about one minute per side.
3. Stir together the rest of the ingredients and then pour over the scallops in the pot.
4. Cover and lock the pot.
5. Using the Pressure setting, set the cook time for 2 minutes.
6. At the end of the cook time, carefully vent the pot manually.
7. Serve the scallops drizzled with sauce from the pot.

Nutrition Information Per Serving:

- Total Fat: 6 grams
- Carbohydrates: 26 grams
- Protein: 25 grams

Vegan and Vegetarian

Meat, poultry and fish are a big part of most diets because they're the most reliable sources of protein, but it's also possible to use the Ninja Foodi to prepare vegetarian dishes that satisfy the requirements of a nutrition plan that excludes meat. The recipes in this section are all vegetarian, and some them are vegan-friendly, as well. They include main dishes, vegetable side dishes and desserts.

Ninja Foodi Cauliflower Curry

Servings: 6
Time Required: About 25 minutes
Ingredients:

- 1 head cauliflower, chopped
- ½ onion, chopped
- 2 tomatoes, chopped
- 6 cloves garlic, minced
- 1 Tbsp. fresh ginger, peeled and minced
- ½ jalapeno chili, diced
- 1 tsp. olive oil
- ½ tsp. turmeric
- 1 tsp. ground cumin
- ½ tsp. garam masala
- ¾ tsp. salt
- ½ tsp. paprika

Method:

1. Place onion, tomato, chili, ginger and garlic in a blender or food processor and blend until smooth.
2. Push Saute button on the Ninja Foodi and add oil. When the oil is hot, add mixture from the blender to the pot.
3. Add the spices to the pot and stir to mix. Cover the pot and allow to cook for 5 minutes.
4. Stir the cauliflower into the pot and then close and lock the pot. Press the Keep Warm button to stop the Sauté cycle.
5. Using the Pressure mode, set the cook time for 2 minutes.
6. At the end of the cook time, carefully vent the pot manually.
7. Serve hot.

Nutrition Information Per Serving:

- Total Fat: 1 gram
- Carbohydrates: 20 grams
- Protein: 4 grams

Ninja Foodi Mexican-Style Mushrooms

Servings: 2
Time Required: About 30 minutes
Ingredients:

- 8 oz. white mushrooms, chopped
- 2 large chili peppers, such as guajillo, poblano or New Mexico, seeded and chopped
- 1 tsp. olive oil
- 1 onion, chopped
- 6 cloves garlic, minced
- 1 tsp. ground cumin
- ½ tsp. dried oregano
- ½ tsp. smoked paprika
- ¼ tsp. ground cinnamon
- ¼ tsp. salt
- ¼ cup water
- 1 tsp. cider vinegar

Method:

1. Press the Sauté button on the pot and add oil. When the oil is hot, add the onions to the pot and sauté until soft and translucent, about 5 minutes.
2. Add garlic to the pot and sauté for one minute more.
3. Transfer half of the onion and garlic to a blender or food processor.
4. Add mushrooms to the pot and cook for 5 minutes more.
5. Meanwhile, add chilis to the blender or food processor. Add cumin, oregano, paprika, cinnamon, salt and water. Blend until smooth.
6. Transfer the blended sauce mixture to the Ninja Foodi.
7. Cover and lock the pot and stop the Sauté cycle.
8. Using the Pressure mode, set cook time for 5 minutes.
9. At the end of the cook time, carefully vent the pot manually.
10. Serve the mushrooms hot with steamed cauliflower.

Nutrition Information Per Serving:

- Total Fat: 12 grams
- Carbohydrates: 16 grams
- Protein: 4 grams

Ninja Foodi Green Chili Bake

Servings: 4
Time Required: About 45 minutes
Ingredients:

- 4 eggs, beaten
- 1 cup half and half
- 10 oz. canned green chilis
- ½ tsp. salt
- ½ tsp. ground cumin
- 1 cup Monterey Jack cheese, grated
- ¼ cup fresh cilantro, chopped

Method:

1. In a medium bowl, combine eggs, half and half, chilis, cheese, salt and cumin.
2. Pour the mixture into a greased pan that's small enough to fit into your Ninja Foodi. Cover the pan with aluminum foil.
3. Place the steamer rack into the Ninja Foodi and pour in 2 cups of water.
4. Place the pan on top of the steamer rack.
5. Cover and lock the pot.
6. Using the Pressure mode, cook for 20 minutes.
7. After the cooking time ends, allow the pot to vent naturally for 10 minutes. After 10 minutes, carefully vent any remaining steam and uncover the pot.
8. Remove the pan from the pot and allow to cool slightly before serving.

Nutrition Information Per Serving:

Total Fat: 19 grams
Carbohydrates: 6 grams
Protein: 14 grams

Ninja Foodi Indian Eggplant

Servings: 4
Time Required: About 30 minutes
Ingredients:

- 1 medium eggplant, peeled and sliced
- 1/3 cup olive oil
- 3 cloves garlic, minced
- ½ onion, chopped
- ¼ tsp. turmeric
- 1/8 tsp. cayenne pepper
- ½ tsp. salt
- 1/3 cup tomatoes, diced
- ½ cup water
- 2 Tbsp. fresh cilantro, chopped

Method:

1. Press the Sauté button on the Ninja Foodi and heat 2 tablespoons of the olive oil in the pot. Once the oil is hot, add enough eggplant slices to cover the bottom of the pot liner. Allow the eggplant to brown well on the bottom, and add more eggplant as the slices shrink. Add more oil as necessary.
2. When the eggplant is browned and softened, add the onions and sauté for 5 minutes more.
3. Add the garlic and sauté for another minute.
4. Add the turmeric, cayenne, and salt. Sauté until fragrant, about a minute.
5. Add the tomatoes and water, and stir to combine everything in the pot.
6. Stop the Sauté cycle and cover and lock the pot.
7. Using the Pressure mode, cook for 3 minutes.
8. At the end of the cooking time, carefully vent the pot manually.
9. Uncover the pot and transfer the eggplant and sauce to a serving platter.
10. Serve hot, garnished with cilantro.

Nutrition Information Per Serving:

Total Fat: 12 grams
Carbohydrates: 6 grams
Protein: 1 gram

Ninja Foodi Palak Paneer

Servings: 4
Time Required: About 25 minutes
Ingredients:

- 1 lb. fresh spinach
- 1 ½ cups paneer
- 2 tsp. olive oil
- 5 cloves garlic, minced
- 1 Tbsp. fresh ginger, peeled and minced
- 1 onion, chopped
- 2 tomatoes, chopped
- 2 tsp. ground cumin
- ½ tsp. cayenne pepper
- 2 tsp. garam masala
- 1 tsp. turmeric
- 1 tsp. salt
- ½ cup water

Method:

1. Press the Sauté button on the pot and add oil. When the oil is hot, add the garlic and ginger and sauté just until fragrant, about 30 seconds.
2. Add the rest of the ingredients, excluding the paneer, and stir to combine.
3. Cover and lock the pot and stop the Sauté cycle.
4. Using the Pressure mode, set the cook time for 4 minutes.
5. At the end of the cook time, allow the pot to vent naturally for 10 minutes.
6. After 10 minutes, carefully vent any remaining steam and uncover the pot.
7. Carefully add the paneer to the pot, stirring gently to combine.
8. Serve hot.

Nutrition Information Per Serving:

- Total Fat: 16 grams
- Carbohydrates: 8 grams
- Protein: 11 grams

Ninja Foodi Low-Carb Cake

Servings: 4
Time Required: About 1.5 hours
Ingredients:
- 1 cup almond flour
- ½ cup unsweetened coconut, shredded
- 1/3 cup Stevia sweetener
- 1 tsp. baking powder
- ½ tsp. cinnamon
- 2 eggs, lightly beaten
- ¼ cup butter, melted
- ½ cup heavy whipping cream

Method:
1. In a medium bowl, combine almond flour, coconut, sweetener, baking powder and cinnamon.
2. Whisk in eggs, butter and cream, one at a time, until all ingredients are well combined.
3. Pour the mixture into a pan that's small enough to fit into your Ninja Foodi. Cover the pan with foil.
4. Place the steamer rack into the Ninja Foodi and pour in 2 cups of water.
5. Place the pan onto the steamer rack.
6. Cover and lock the pot.
7. Using the Pressure mode, set the cook time for 40 minutes.
8. At the end of the cook time, allow the pot to vent naturally for 10 minutes.
9. After 10 minutes, carefully release any remaining steam and uncover the pot.
10. Remove the pan from the pot and allow to cool for 15 minutes. After the cake has cooled, flip the pan over and carefully encourage the cake out of the pan.

Nutrition Information Per Serving:
- Total Fat: 23 grams
- Carbohydrates: 5 grams
- Protein: 5 grams

Ninja Foodi Carrot Cake

Servings: 4
Time Required: About 1.5 hours
Ingredients:

- 3 eggs
- 1 cup almond flour
- 2/3 cup Stevia-based sweetener
- 1 tsp. baking powder
- ½ Tbsp. apple pie spice
- ¼ cup coconut oil
- ½ cup heavy cream
- 1 cup carrots, shredded
- ½ cup walnuts, chopped

Method:

1. In a medium mixing bowl, mix all the ingredients using an electric mixer until the batter is well-mixed and fluffy.
2. Pour batter into a greased cake pan that's small enough to fit into your Ninja Foodi. Cover the pan with aluminum foil.
3. Place the steamer rack in the Ninja Foodi and pour in 2 cups of water.
4. Place the pan on the steamer rack.
5. Cover and lock the pot.
6. Using the Pressure mode, cook for 40 minutes.
7. At the end of the cooking cycle, allow the pot to vent naturally for 10 minutes. After 10 minutes, carefully vent any remaining pressure and uncover the pot.
8. Remove the pan from the pot and allow the cake to cool before serving.

Nutrition Information Per Serving:

- Total Fat: 25 grams
- Carbohydrates: 6 grams
- Protein: 6 grams

Ninja Foodi Coconut Cake

Servings: 4
Time Required: About 1.5 hours
Ingredients:

- 1 cup almond flour
- ½ cup unsweetened coconut, shredded
- 1/3 cup Stevia-based sweetener
- 1 tsp. baking powder
- 1 tsp. apple pie spice
- 2 eggs
- ¼ cup butter, softened
- ½ cup heavy cream

Method:

1. In a medium mixing bowl, mix all the ingredients using an electric mixer until the batter is well-mixed and fluffy.
2. Pour batter into a greased cake pan that's small enough to fit into your Ninja Foodi. Cover the pan with aluminum foil.
3. Place the steamer rack in the Ninja Foodi and pour in 2 cups of water.
4. Place the pan on the steamer rack.
5. Cover and lock the pot.
6. Using the Pressure mode, cook for 40 minutes.
7. At the end of the cooking cycle, allow the pot to vent naturally for 10 minutes. After 10 minutes, carefully vent any remaining pressure and uncover the pot.
8. Remove the pan from the pot and allow the cake to cool before serving.

Nutrition Information Per Serving:

- Total Fat: 23 grams
- Carbohydrates: 5 grams
- Protein: 5 grams

Ninja Foodi Cheesecake

Servings: 4
Time Required: About 9.5 hours
Ingredients:

- 16 oz. cream cheese
- ½ cup low-carb sweetener
- ½ tsp. vanilla extract
- Zest of 1 lemon
- 3 eggs
- ¼ cup heavy cream
- ½ cup sour cream

Method:

1. Use an electric mixer to combine cream cheese, sweetener, heavy cream, vanilla and lemon zest. Add eggs one at a time, mixing just enough to combine.
2. Pour the mixture into a lightly greased cake pan that's small enough to fit into your Ninja Foodi. Cover the pan with aluminum foil.
3. Place the steamer rack into the Ninja Foodi and pour in 2 cups of water.
4. Place the covered pan on top of the steamer rack. Cover and lock the pot.
5. Using the Pressure mode, cook for 40 minutes.
6. At the end of the cooking time, allow the pot to vent naturally for 15 minutes. After 15 minutes, carefully vent any remaining pressure and uncover the pot.
7. Remove the pan and spread the sour cream evenly over the top of the cheesecake.
8. Refrigerate the cheesecake for at least 8 hours.
9. When the cheesecake is cooled, spoon into serving bowls.

Nutrition Information Per Serving:

- Total Fat: 24 grams
- Carbohydrates: 3 grams
- Protein: 7 grams

Side Dishes

Your Ninja Foodi can do more than just prepare each meal's main dish. The recipes in this section give you side dishes that add depth and variety to your balanced meals.

Ninja Foodi Garlic Zucchini Fries

Servings: 6
Time Required: About 25 minutes
Ingredients:

- 4 large zucchini, sliced into fries of desired thickness
- 4 Tbsp. butter, melted
- 2 Tbsp. garlic, minced
- 2 Tbsp. chopped fresh parsely
- 3 Tbsp. freshly grated Parmesan cheese
- ½ cup water

Method:

1. Place zucchini into the Air Crisp basket, and place the basket in the pot.
2. Combine the butter, chopped garlic, parsley, and cheese in a small bowl.
3. Pour the butter mixture over fries and close the crisping lid.
4. Set to Air Crisp at 400 degrees for 12 minutes.
5. After 5 minutes, carefully stir the fries to keep them from sticking.
6. Continue to cook, checking often, until the fries are crisp and golden brown.

Nutrition Information Per Serving

- Total Fat: 4 grams
- Carbohydrates: 1 gram
- Protein: 4 grams

Ninja Foodi Bacon Brussels Sprouts

Servings: 4
Time Required: About 30 minutes
Ingredients:

- 24 oz. Brussels sprouts, cut in half
- 3 Tbsp. bacon fat or butter
- ¼ cup chopped onion
- 1 Tbsp. garlic, minced
- ½ tsp. garlic powder

Method:

1. Using the sauté mode, sauté onion, garlic, sprouts and seasonings in the Foodi, stirring constantly, until the onions are translucent.
2. Remove the mixture from the Foodi and set aside. Carefully wipe the pot clean.
3. Add half the seasoned Brussels sprouts to the Air Crisp basket, place the basket in the pot.
4. Set to Air Crisp at 390 degrees for 12 minutes. Cook until the sprouts are crispy.
5. Remove to a plate and season with salt.
6. Repeat with the rest of the Brussels sprouts.

Nutrition Information Per Serving:

- Total Fat: 8 grams
- Carbohydrates: 3 grams
- Protein: 3 grams

Ninja Foodi Artichokes

Servings: 4

Time Required: About 35 minutes

Ingredients:

- 4 artichokes, medium-sized
- 1 lemon
- 4 cups vegetable stock
- ¼ tsp. kosher salt

Method:

1. Trim the artichoke stems to an inch in length. Trim the other end of the artichokes, too, cutting the inch from the ends of the leaves. Discard the trimmings.
2. Slice the lemon into four slices.
3. Place the steamer rack into the Ninja Foodi and place the lemon slices on the rack. Place the artichokes, stem end up, on the lemon slices, one artichoke on each lemon slice.
4. Pour the stock carefully into the pot. Season with salt.
5. Cover and lock the pot.
6. Using the Pressure mode, set the cook time for 20 minutes and start the cook cycle.
7. At the end of the cooking time, carefully vent the pot manually and remove the cover.
8. Serve the artichokes with melted butter for dipping.

Nutrition Information Per Serving:

- Total Fat: 1 gram
- Carbohydrates: 13 grams
- Protein: 4 grams

Ninja Foodi Cheese and Cauliflower Casserole

Servings: 6
Time Required: About 45 minutes
Ingredients

- 1 head cauliflower
- 2 eggs
- 2 Tbsp. heavy cream
- 2 oz. cream cheese
- ½ cup sour cream
- ½ cup Parmesan cheese, grated
- 1 cup cheddar cheese, grated
- 2 Tbsp. butter
- 1 cup water

Method:

1. Add eggs, cream, sour cream, cream cheese, Parmesan and cheddar cheese to a blender or food processor. Blend to combine.
2. Add cauliflower to the food processor and blend, pulsing so that you can stop when the mixture is still chunky, not smooth.
3. Grease a casserole pan that's small enough to fit in your Ninja Foodi and pour the mixture into the pan.
4. Place the steamer rack into the Ninja Foodi and pour in a cup of water.
5. Place the casserole pan on the steamer rack.
6. Cover and lock the pot.
7. Using the Pressure mode, set the cook time for 12 minutes.
8. At the end of the cook time, allow the pot to vent naturally for 10 minutes.
9. After 10 minutes, carefully vent any remaining steam and uncover the pot.
10. Remove the pan and serve the casserole hot.

Nutrition Information Per Serving:

- Total Fat: 28 grams
- Carbohydrates: 7 grams
- Protein: 17 grams

Ninja Foodi Basic Spaghetti Squash

Servings: 4
Time Required: About 25 minutes
Ingredients:
- 1 spaghetti squash, medium
- 1 cup water

Method:
1. With a sharp knife, carefully cut the squash in half crosswise, across the short length of the squash instead of along the longer axis.
2. Use a metal spoon to scoop the seeds and loose flesh out of the center of both halves of the squash.
3. Put the steamer rack into the Ninja Foodi and pour in a cup of water.
4. Place the squash halves on the steamer rack, cut side up.
5. Cover and lock the pot.
6. Using the Pressure mode, set the cook time to 7 minutes and start the cook cycle.
7. At the end of the cook time, carefully vent the pot manually and remove the cover.
8. Remove the squash and, while it's still hot, carefully shred the flesh into spaghetti-like strands with a fork.
9. Serve the squash hot with butter.

Nutrition Information Per Serving:
- Total Fat: 1 gram
- Carbohydrates: 7 grams
- Protein: 1 gram

Ninja Foodi Garlic Spaghetti Squash

Servings: 4
Time Required: About 25 minutes
Ingredients:

- 1 medium spaghetti squash
- 1 cup water
- 4 cloves garlic, minced
- 1 Tbsp. olive oil
- 1 tsp. salt
- 1/8 tsp. nutmeg

Method:

1. With a sharp knife, carefully cut the squash in half crosswise, across the short length of the squash instead of along the longer axis.
2. Use a metal spoon to scoop the seeds and loose flesh out of the center of both halves of the squash.
3. Put the steamer rack into the Ninja Foodi and pour in a cup of water.
4. Place the squash halves on the steamer rack, cut side up.
5. Cover and lock the pot.
6. Using the Pressure mode, set the cook time to 7 minutes and start the cook cycle.
7. At the end of the cook time, carefully vent the pot manually and remove the cover.
8. Remove the squash and, while it's still hot, carefully shred the flesh into spaghetti-like strands with a fork.
9. Empty and dry the Ninja Foodi liner and put it back into the pot.
10. Press the Sauté button on the Ninja Foodi and add the oil. When the oil is hot, add the garlic and sauté just until fragrant, about 30 seconds.
11. Toss the garlic, salt and nutmeg with the shredded squash and serve hot. For an extra kick of flavor, sprinkle with freshly grated Parmesan cheese.

Nutrition Information Per Serving:

- Total Fat: 4 grams
- Carbohydrates: 13 grams
- Protein: 2 grams

Ninja Foodi Cauliflower Mash

Servings: 6
Time Required: About 15 minutes
Ingredients:

- 1 head cauliflower
- 1/8 tsp. salt
- 1/8 tsp. freshly ground black pepper
- ¼ tsp. garlic powder
- 1 cup water

Method:

1. Chop the cauliflower coarsely and discard the tough core.
2. Place the steamer rack in the Ninja Foodi and add a cup of water.
3. Place the cauliflower on top of the steamer rack.
4. Cover and lock the pot.
5. Using the Pressure mode, set the cook time to 4 minutes.
6. At the end of the cooking time, carefully vent the pot manually. Uncover the pot.
7. Remove the pot liner and carefully drain the water and remove the steamer rack, returning the cauliflower to the pot once it's drained.
8. If you have an immersion blender, use it to blend the cauliflower to a smooth puree, adding the seasonings as you blend. If you don't have an immersion blender, transfer the cauliflower to a blender or food processor. Optionally, you can add a tablespoon of butter as you blend for a creamier consistency.
9. Serve hot.

Nutrition Information Per Serving:

- Total Fat: 1 gram
- Carbohydrates: 5 grams
- Protein: 2 grams

Ninja Foodi Coconut Cabbage

Servings: 6
Time Required: About 20 minutes
Ingredients:

- 1 Tbsp. olive oil
- 1 medium onion, sliced
- 1 tsp. salt
- 2 cloves garlic, minced
- ½ Thai red chili, seeded and sliced
- 1 tsp. dry mustard
- 1 Tbsp. curry powder
- 1 Tbsp. turmeric powder
- 1 Asian cabbage, cored and shredded
- 1 carrot, peeled and sliced
- 2 lemon juice
- ½ cup dried unsweetened coconut, shredded
- 1/3 cup water

Method:

1. Press the Sauté button on the pot and add oil. When the oil is hot, sauté the onions until they are soft and translucent, about 5 minutes.
2. Add garlic, chili pepper and spices and sauté for about 30 seconds more, just until fragrant.
3. Add the cabbage, carrot, lemon juice and water, stirring to combine.
4. Cover and lock the pot, and stop the Sauté cycle.
5. Using the Pressure mode, set the cook time to 5 minutes.
6. At the end of the cooking time, carefully vent the pot manually.
7. Remove the cover and serve the cabbage hot as a side dish.

Nutrition Information Per Serving:

- Total Fat: 1 gram
- Carbohydrates: 6 grams
- Protein: 1 gram

Ninja Foodi Garlic Zucchini

Servings: 4
Time Required: About 15 minutes
Ingredients:

- 2 large zucchini, peeled and coarsely grated
- 2 Tbsp. olive oil
- 2 cloves garlic, minced
- 1 tsp. lemon zest
- ½ tsp. sea salt
- 1 Tbsp. fresh lemon juice
- Salt and pepper to taste

Method:

1. Press the Sauté button on the pot and add oil. When the oil is hot, sauté the garlic and lemon zest just until fragrant, about 30 seconds.
2. Add the zucchini and season to taste with salt and pepper. Sprinkle lemon juice over the top of the zucchini.
3. Sauté, stirring, just until zucchini is heated through, about 2 or 3 minutes.
4. Remove from the pot and serve hot.

Nutrition Information Per Serving:

- Total Fat: 1 gram
- Carbohydrates: 4 grams
- Protein: 1 gram

Ninja Foodi Egg Salad

Servings: 6
Time Required: About 35 minutes
Ingredients:

- 10 eggs
- 5 slices bacon
- 2 Tbsp. mayonnaise
- 1 tsp. Dijon mustard
- ¼ tsp. smoked paprika
- 1 spring onion, diced
- Salt and pepper to taste

Method:

1. Crack the eggs and place them in a greased pan that's small enough to fit into your Ninja Foodi.
2. Place the steamer rack into the Ninja Foodi and pour in a cup of water. Place the pan with the eggs on top of the steamer rack.
3. Cover and lock the pot.
4. Using the Pressure mode, set the cook time for 6 minutes and start the cook cycle.
5. At the end of the cooking time, allow the pot to vent naturally for 10 minutes.
6. After 10 minutes, carefully vent any remaining steam and uncover the pot.
7. Remove the pan and transfer the cooked eggs to a cutting board. Chop the eggs coarsely and transfer to a mixing bowl.
8. Empty and dry the Ninja Foodi liner and put it back into the pot.
9. Press the Sauté button on the Ninja Foodi. While the pot is heating, coarsely chop the bacon and add it to the pot.
10. Sauté the bacon until it's crispy, then carefully add the bacon and its fat to the chopped eggs.
11. Add the rest of the ingredients to the mixing bowl toss well to combine.
12. Serve garnished with chopped chives.

Nutrition Information Per Serving:

- Total Fat: 26 grams
- Carbohydrates: 2 grams
- Protein: 16 grams

Ninja Foodi Basic Brussels Sprouts

Servings: 4
Time Required: About 15 minutes
Ingredients:

- 4 cups Brussels sprouts, ends trimmed and cut in half
- 1 tsp. olive oil
- ½ cup water
- Salt to taste

Method:

1. Press the Sauté button on the pot and add oil. When the oil is hot, sauté the brussels sprouts, stirring frequently, until the sprouts are beginning to brown and get crisp at the edges. This should take about 5 minutes.
2. When the sprouts are browned, carefully add the water to the pot.
3. Cover and lock the pot and stop the Sauté cycle.
4. Using the Pressure mode, set the cook time to 2 minutes.
5. At the end of the cooking time, carefully vent the pot manually.
6. Remove the cover and season the Brussels sprout with sea salt to taste.
7. Serve hot.

Nutrition Information Per Serving

- Total Fat: 1 gram
- Carbohydrates: 8 grams
- Protein: 3 grams

Ninja Foodi Keema Curry

Servings: 6
Time Required: About 1.25 hours
Ingredients:

- 2 Tbsp. olive oil
- 1 onion, diced
- 4 cloves garlic, minced
- 1 inch piece of fresh ginger, peeled and minced
- 1 Serrano pepper, seeded and minced
- 1 Tbsp. coriander
- 1 tsp. paprika
- 1 tsp. salt
- ½ tsp. turmeric
- ½ tsp. black pepper
- ½ tsp. garam masala
- ½ tsp. cumin powder
- ¼ tsp. cayenne
- ¼ tsp. ground cardamom
- 1 lb. ground beef
- 1 can diced tomatoes
- 2 cups fresh or frozen peas

Method:

1. Press the Sauté button on the pot and add oil. When the oil is hot, sauté the onions until they are beginning to brown, about 8 minutes.
2. Add garlic, ginger, Serrano pepper, and spices, and sauté for about 1 minute more.
3. Add the ground beef and sauté until the meat is thoroughly browned, about 5-10 minutes.
4. Add the tomatoes and peas to the pot, stirring to combine all the ingredients.
5. Cover and lock the pot and stop the Sauté cycle.
6. Using the Pressure mode, set the cook time for 30 minutes.
7. At the end of the cooking time, allow the pot to vent naturally for 10 minutes.
8. After 10 minutes, carefully vent any remaining steam and uncover the pot.
9. Serve the curry hot.

Nutrition Information Per Serving:

- Total Fat: 20 grams
- Carbohydrates: 17 grams
- Protein: 30 grams

Ninja Foodi Creamy Cauliflower with Cheese

Servings: 4
Time Required: About 15 minutes
Ingredients:

- 2 cups cauliflower, riced
- 2 Tbsp. cream cheese
- ½ cup half and half
- ½ cup cheddar cheese, grated
- Salt and Pepper to taste

Method:

1. Combine all the ingredients in a baking dish that's small enough to fit in your Ninja Foodi. Cover the dish with aluminum foil.
2. Put the steamer rack into the Ninja Foodi and pour in a cup of water. Place the baking dish on top of the steamer rack.
3. Using the Pressure mode, set the cook time for 5 minutes and start the cook cycle.
4. At the end of the cooking time, allow the pot to vent naturally for 10 minutes.
5. After 10 minutes, carefully vent any remaining steam and uncover the pot.
6. Remove the baking dish and serve the cooked cauliflower hot.

Nutrition Information Per Serving:

- Total Fat: 10 grams
- Carbohydrates: 4 grams
- Protein: 5 grams

Conclusion

With the time-saving technology of the Ninja Foodi in your hands, you've now got the tools to transform a list of common, healthy ingredients into irresistibly satisfying culinary creations. You don't need anything else to make the changes that will lead you to a healthier lifestyle. There's nothing standing in your way, and the path to a new you starts right here, right now.

CPSIA information can be obtained
at www.ICGtesting.com
Printed in the USA
BVHW010205141119
563818BV00008B/99/P